G000122997

PEDIATRIC DRUG RESEARCH
AND THE FDA

PHARMACOLOGY - RESEARCH, SAFETY TESTING AND REGULATION

Additional books in this series can be found on Nova's website
under the Series tab.

Additional E-books in this series can be found on Nova's website
under the E-book tab.

PHARMACOLOGY - RESEARCH, SAFETY TESTING AND REGULATION

PEDIATRIC DRUG RESEARCH AND THE FDA

KEVIN L. WASHINGTON
AND
JEFF E. BENNETT
EDITORS

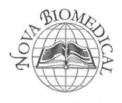

Nova Science Publishers, Inc.

New York

Library of Congress Cataloging-in-Publication Data

ISBN 978-1-62257-729-3

Published by Nova Science Publishers, Inc. † New York

CONTENTS

PREFACE

Congress reauthorized two laws in 2007, the Pediatric Research Equity Act (PREA) and the Best Pharmaceuticals for Children Act (BPCA). PREA requires that sponsors conduct pediatric studies for certain products unless the Department of Health and Human Services' (HHS) Food and Drug Administration (FDA) grants a waiver or deferral. On June 20th, 2012, the House of Representatives passed, by voice vote and under suspension of the rules, the Food and Drug Administration Safety and Innovation Act, as amended. This bill would reauthorize the FDA prescription drug and medical device user fee programs, create new user fee programs for generic and biosimilar drug approvals, and make other revisions to other FDA drug and device approval processes. This book examines how many and what types of products have been studied; describes the number and type of labeling changes and FDA's review periods and describes challenges identified by stakeholders to conducting studies.

Chapter 1 – On June 20, 2012, the House of Representatives passed, by voice vote and under suspension of the rules, S. 3187 (EAH), the Food and Drug Administration Safety and Innovation Act, as amended. This bill would reauthorize the FDA prescription drug and medical device user fee programs (which would otherwise expire on September 30, 2012), create new user fee programs for generic and biosimilar drug approvals, and make other revisions to other FDA drug and device approval processes. It reflects bicameral compromise on earlier versions of the bill (S. 3187 [ES], which passed the Senate on May 24, 2012, and H.R. 5651 [EH], which passed the House on May 30, 2012).

Chaptaer 2 – The FDA Modernization Act of 1997 (FDAMA) established pediatric exclusivity for sponsors that conducted pediatric studies for drugs. In 1999, FDA implemented the Pediatric Rule, which required that sponsors include the results of pediatric studies when submitting certain new drug or biological product applications. However, in 2002, the Pediatric Rule was declared invalid by a federal court. In 2002, Congress reauthorized FDAMA's pediatric exclusivity provisions in BPCA, and in 2003, Congress codified much of the Pediatric Rule in PREA, requiring that pediatric studies be conducted and that the results of those studies be included in certain new drug or biological product applications. In September 2007, Congress reauthorized both PREA and BPCA as a part of FDAAA, and in March 2010, Congress extended pediatric exclusivity and applicable BPCA provisions to biological products as a part of the Patient Protection and Affordable Care Act. PREA and BPCA are both set to expire on October 1, 2012.

In: Pediatric Drug Research and the FDA   ISBN 978-1-62257-729-3
Editors: K. Washington and J. Bennett   © 2013 Nova Science Publishers, Inc.

Chapter 1

FDA'S AUTHORITY TO ENSURE THAT DRUGS PRESCRIBED TO CHILDREN ARE SAFE AND EFFECTIVE[*]

Susan Thaul

On June 20, 2012, the House of Representatives passed, by voice vote and under suspension of the rules, S. 3187 (EAH), the Food and Drug Administration Safety and Innovation Act, as amended. This bill would reauthorize the FDA prescription drug and medical device user fee programs (which would otherwise expire on September 30, 2012), create new user fee programs for generic and biosimilar drug approvals, and make other revisions to other FDA drug and device approval processes. It reflects bicameral compromise on earlier versions of the bill (S. 3187 [ES], which passed the Senate on May 24, 2012, and H.R. 5651 [EH], which passed the House on May 30, 2012).

SUMMARY

With the Best Pharmaceuticals for Children Act (BPCA) and the Pediatric Research Equity Act (PREA), Congress authorized the Food and Drug

---

[*] This is an edited, reformatted and augmented version of the Congressional Research Service Publication, CRS Report for Congress RL33986, dated June 25, 2012.

Administration (FDA) to offer drug manufacturers financial and regulatory incentives to test their products for use in children. Congress extended both programs with the FDA Amendments of 2007 (FDAAA) and, because of the programs' sunset date, must act before October 1, 2012, to continue them. This report presents the historical development of BPCA and PREA, their rationale and effect, and FDAAA's impact. The report also discusses pediatric drug issues that remain of concern to some in Congress.

Most prescription drugs have never been the subject of studies specifically designed to test their effects on children. In these circumstances, clinicians, therefore, may prescribe drugs for children that FDA has approved only for adult use; this practice is known as off-label prescribing. Although some clinicians may believe that the safety and effectiveness demonstrated with adults would hold for younger patients, studies show that the bioavailability of drugs—that is, how much gets into a patient's system and is available for use—varies in children for reasons that include a child's maturation and organ development and other factors. The result of such off-label prescribing may be that some children receive ineffective drugs or too much or too little of potentially useful drugs; or that there may be side effects unique to children, including effects on growth and development.

Drug manufacturers are reluctant to test drugs in children because of economic, ethical, legal, and other obstacles. Market forces alone have not provided manufacturers with sufficient incentives to overcome these obstacles. BPCA and PREA represent attempts by Congress to address the need for pediatric testing. FDA had tried unsuccessfully to spur pediatric drug research through administrative action before 1997. With the FDA Modernization Act of 1997 (FDAMA, P.L. 105-115), Congress provided an incentive: if a manufacturer completed pediatric studies that FDA requested, the agency would extend the company's market exclusivity for that product for six months, not approving the sale of another manufacturer's product during that period. In 2002, BPCA (P.L. 107-109) reauthorized this program for five years.

In 1998, to obtain pediatric use information on the drugs that manufacturers were not studying, FDA published the Pediatric Rule, which required manufacturers to submit pediatric testing data at the time of all new drug applications. In 2002, a federal court declared the rule invalid, holding that FDA lacked the statutory authority to promulgate it. Congress gave FDA that authority with PREA (P.L. 108-155). PREA covers drugs and biological products and includes provisions for deferrals, waivers, and the required pediatric assessment of an approved marketed product.

In extending BPCA and PREA in 2007, Congress considered several issues: Why offer a financial incentive to encourage pediatric studies when FDA has the authority to require them? How does the cost of marketing exclusivity—including the higher prices paid by government—compare with the cost of the needed research? What percentage of labeling includes pediatric information because of BPCA and PREA? Do existing laws provide FDA with sufficient authority to encourage pediatric studies and labeling? Is FDA doing enough with its current authority? The 112th Congress will likely consider those questions as well as others: What information do clinicians and consumers need and how could industry and government develop and disseminate it? How can Congress balance positive and negative incentives to manufacturers for developing pediatric information to use in labeling? How could Congress consider cost and benefit when it deals with reauthorizing legislation in 2012?

INTRODUCTION

The Food and Drug Administration (FDA) has approved for adult use many drugs that have been tested for adults but not for children. Yet clinicians often prescribe adult-approved drugs for children, a practice known as off-label prescribing, (1) because most drugs have not been tested in children,[1] and (2) because clinicians presume that the safety and effectiveness demonstrated with adults generally means that the drugs are also safe and effective for children. However, research shows, as described later in this report and in **Table 1**, that this is not always true. Children may need higher or lower doses than adults, may experience effects on their growth and development, and may not respond to drugs approved for adults.

Congress passed the Best Pharmaceuticals for Children Act (BPCA) of 2002 and the Pediatric Research Equity Act (PREA) of 2003 to encourage drug manufacturers to develop and label drugs for pediatric use.[2] BPCA offers manufacturers incentives to conduct pediatric-specific research. PREA requires certain pediatric use information in products' labeling.[3] The Food and Drug Administration Amendments Act of 2007 (FDAAA, P.L. 110-85)[4] reauthorized and strengthened the programs' authorizing legislation. The FDAAA authority for these two programs is set to end on October 1, 2012, unless Congress reauthorizes the efforts.

This report describes how and why Congress developed these initiatives. Specifically, the report

- describes why research on a drug's pharmacokinetics, safety, and effectiveness in children might be necessary;
- presents why the marketplace has not provided sufficient incentives to manufacturers of drugs approved for adult use to study their effects in children;
- describes how BPCA provides extended market exclusivity in return for FDA-requested studies on pediatric use, and how PREA requires studies of drugs' safety and effectiveness when used by children (**Appendix B** analyzes how BPCA and PREA evolved from FDA's administrative earlier efforts);
- analyzes the impact BPCA and PREA have had on pediatric drug research; and
- discusses issues, some of which Congress considered leading up to FDAAA, that may form the basis of oversight and evaluative activities along with reauthorization efforts in 2012.

UNDERSTANDING DRUG EFFECTS IN CHILDREN

A drug cannot be marketed in the United States without FDA approval. A manufacturer's application to FDA must include an "Indication for Use" section that describes what the drug does as well as the clinical condition and population for which the manufacturer has done the testing and for which it seeks approval for sale.

To approve a drug, FDA must determine that the manufacturer has sufficiently demonstrated the drug's safety and effectiveness for the intended indication[5] and population specified in the application.[6] The Federal Food, Drug, and Cosmetic Act[7] (FFDCA) allows a manufacturer to promote or advertise a drug only for uses listed in the FDA-approved labeling—and the labeling may list only those claims for which FDA has reviewed and accepted safety and effectiveness evidence.

Once FDA approves a drug, a licensed physician may—except in highly regulated circumstances—prescribe it without restriction.[8] When a clinician prescribes a drug to an individual whose demographic or medical characteristics differ from those indicated in a drug's FDA-approved labeling, that is called *off-label use*, which is considered accepted medical practice.

Most prescriptions that physicians write for children fall into the category of off-label use. In these instances, because FDA has not been presented with data relating to the drugs' use in children, no labeling information is included to address indications, dosage, or warnings related to use in children. Faced with an ill child, a clinician must decide whether the drug might help. The doctor must also decide what dose and how often the drug should be taken, all to best balance the drug's intended effect with its anticipated and unanticipated side effects.

Such clinicians face an obstacle: children are not miniature adults.[9] At different ages, a body may handle a given amount of an administered drug differently, resulting in varying bioavailability. This occurs, in part, because the rate at which the body eliminates a drug (after which the drug is no longer present) varies, among other things, according to changes in the maturation and development of organs. Clearance (elimination from the body) can be quicker or slower in children, depending on the age of child, the organs involved, and body surface area.[10]

Table 1. Examples of Differences in Effectiveness, Dosing, and Adverse Events for Children Administered Adult-Tested, FDA-Approved Medications

Type of difference	Example of drug demonstrating this difference
Inability to demonstrate effectiveness	• some cancer drugs • buspirone (Buspar) for general anxiety disorder • some combination diabetes drugs
Children require higher doses than adults	• gabapentin (Neurontin) for seizures: in children less than 5 years old • fluvoxamine (Luvox) for obsessive compulsive disorder (OCD): in adolescents (12- to 17-year-olds) • benazepril (Lotensin) for hypertension
Children require lower doses than adults	• famotidine (Pepcid) for gastroesophageal reflux: in patients less than 3 months of age • fluvoxamine (Luvox) for OCD: in 8- to 11-year-old girls
Unique pediatric adverse events	• betamethasone (Diprolene AF, Lotrisone) for some dermatoses: not recommended in patients less than 12 years of age due to hypopituitary adrenal (HPA) axis suppression
Effects on growth and development	• atomoxetine (Strattera) for attention deficit hyperactivity disorder • fluoxetine (Prozac) for depression and OCD • ribaviron/intron A (Rebetron) for chronic hepatitis C

Sources: Presentations by FDA scientists Dianne Murphy and William Rodriguez, 2006.

FDA scientists have described how drugs act differently in children, noting the kinds of unsatisfactory results that can occur when drugs are prescribed without the pediatric-specific information. These results include unnecessary exposure to ineffective drugs; ineffective dosing of an effective drug; overdosing of an effective drug; undefined unique pediatric adverse events; and effects on growth and behavior.[11] **Table 1** includes examples of drugs for which research has identified different responses between children and adults.

Such examples illustrate why some in Congress believe in the value of conducting studies in children of a drug's pharmacokinetics—the uptake, distribution, binding, elimination, and biotransformation rates within the body. Such studies can help determine whether children need larger or smaller doses than adults. They can also establish whether doses should differ among children of different ages. Clinicians could use pediatric-specific information in the FDA-approved labeling of drugs to help them decide which, if any, drug to use; in what amount; and by what route to administer the drug. Furthermore, well-designed, -conducted, and -disseminated studies in children can reveal information about potential adverse events, thereby allowing clinicians and patients' family members to make better decisions.

WHY MANUFACTURERS HAVE NOT TESTED MOST DRUGS IN CHILDREN

Most drugs—65%-80%—have not been tested in children.[12] Manufacturers face many obstacles—economic, mechanical, ethical, and legal—that make them reluctant to conduct these tests.

The market for any individual drug's pediatric indications is generally small, resulting in a relative economic disincentive for manufacturers to commit resources to pediatric testing compared to drugs for adults. Because young children cannot swallow tablets, a manufacturer might have a mechanical hurdle in developing a different formulation (such as a liquid). The existing ethical and legal requirements encountered in recruiting adult participants for clinical trials may present even greater obstacles when researchers recruit children. Specifically, both the Department of Health and Human Services (HHS) and FDA have issued regulations concerning the protection of human subjects and direct particular attention to the inclusion and protection of vulnerable subjects such as children[13] (see textbox).

Recruiting pediatric study subjects can be difficult because many parents do not want their children in experiments. Also, drug manufacturers face liability concerns that include not only injury but difficult-to-calculate lifetime compensation, made even more difficult regarding a child whose earning potential has not yet been established.

FDA AND THE PROTECTION OF CHILDREN IN CLINICAL RESEARCH

FDA has established certain principles and guidelines regarding child participation in research on FDA-regulated products. Regulations address the need to minimize risk, specifying considerations in different situations, such as when the research involves "greater than minimal risk but presenting the prospect of direct benefit to individual subjects" (21 C.F.R. 50.52); "greater than minimal risk and no prospect of direct benefit to individual subjects, but likely to yield generalizable knowledge about the subjects' disorder or condition" (21 C.F.R. 50.53); and "investigations not otherwise approvable that present an opportunity to understand, prevent, or alleviate a serious problem affecting the health or welfare of children" (21 C.F.R. 50.54).

In a 2008 presentation to the Pediatric Ethics Subcommittee of the FDA Pediatric Advisory Committee, pediatric ethicist Robert Nelson from the FDA Office of Pediatric Therapeutics described the "'nested' protections" of scientific necessity, parental permission, child assent, and appropriate balance of risk and benefit. Dr. Nelson presented the "principle of scientific necessity: Children should not be enrolled in a clinical investigation unless absolutely necessary to answer an important scientific question about the health and welfare of children."

Sources: 21 C.F.R. 50 Part D; and Robert M. Nelson, Pediatric Ethicist, FDA Office of Pediatric Therapeutics, "21 C.F.R. 50, Subpart D: Additional Safeguards for Children in Clinical Investigations of FDA-Regulated Products," presentation to the Pediatric Ethics Subcommittee of the FDA Pediatric Advisory Committee, June 9, 2008, http://www.fda.gov/ohrms/dockets/ac/08/slides/2008-4399s1-13%20%28Nelson%20Presentation%29.pdf.

Congress has offered incentives to manufacturers for pediatric research for two main reasons. First, doctors prescribe drugs approved for adults despite insufficient pediatric-use studies. Second, enough Members of Congress have believed that, despite the difficulty in conducting such studies, children could be better served once the research was done.

BPCA AND PREA: LAWS TO ENCOURAGE PEDIATRIC DRUG RESEARCH

Although Congress has designed other laws (such as those affecting drug development, safety and effectiveness efforts, and general health care and consumer protection) to promote or protect the health of the entire population (including children), the Best Pharmaceuticals for Children Act and the Pediatric Research Equity Act (both sections of the Federal Food, Drug, and Cosmetic Act) authorize programs focused specifically on pediatric drug research. Congress first enacted BPCA and PREA in late 2002 and early 2003, respectively. In 2007, Congress authorized their continuation for another five years.[14]

When presenting information about the pediatric research provisions in law, more than one FDA representative has referred to "the carrot and the stick."[15] BPCA offers a carrot—extending market exclusivity in return for specific studies on pediatric use—and PREA provides a stick— requiring studies of a drug's safety and effectiveness when used by children. This section describes BPCA and PREA and compares them on key dimensions.

Best Pharmaceuticals for Children Act

LEGISLATIVE HISTORY OF BPCA

Congress enacted the current BPCA provisions in three separate pieces of legislation:

- the Better Pharmaceuticals for Children Act, enacted in the FDA Modernization Act of 1997 (FDAMA);
- the Best Pharmaceuticals for Children Act of 2002; and
- the Best Pharmaceuticals for Children Act of 2007, enacted in the FDA Amendments Act of 2007 (FDAAA).

See **Appendix B** for a discussion of the chronological development of BPCA and PREA.

This section covers the main provisions in the Best Pharmaceuticals for Children Act. The law addresses two circumstances: (1) when a drug is on-patent and a manufacturer might benefit from pediatric marketing exclusivity and (2) when a drug is off-patent or a manufacturer does not want additional marketing exclusivity.

Pediatric Marketing Exclusivity

For drugs that are under market exclusivity based on patents or other intact extensions,[16] FFDCA Section 505A (21 U.S.C. 355a) gives FDA the authority to offer manufacturers[17] an additional six-month period of marketing exclusivity in return for FDA-requested pediatric use studies (including preclinical studies) and reports.[18] Marketing exclusivity extends the time before which FDA grants marketing approval for a generic version of the drug. The provision applies to both new drugs and drugs already on the market (except a drug whose other exclusivity is set to expire in less than nine months).

Before FDA sends a manufacturer a written request for pediatric studies, the law requires that an internal review committee, composed of FDA employees with specified expertise, review the request. It also requires that the internal review committee, with the Secretary, track pediatric studies and labeling changes. In addition, it establishes a dispute resolution process, which must include referral to the agency's Pediatric Advisory Committee.

Exclusivity is granted only after (1) a manufacturer completes and reports on the studies that the Secretary had requested in writing, (2) the studies include appropriate formulations of the drug for each age group of interest, and (3) any appropriate labeling changes are approved—all within the agreed upon time frames. The law requires that the manufacturer propose pediatric labeling resulting from the studies. A manufacturer must provide supporting evidence when declining a request for studies on the grounds that developing appropriate pediatric formulations of the drug is not possible.

Applicants for pediatric marketing exclusivity must submit, along with the report of requested studies, all postmarket adverse event reports regarding that drug. The law also has several public notice requirements for the Secretary, including the following:

- notice of exclusivity decisions, along with copies of the written requests;
- public identification of any drug with a developed pediatric formulation that studies had shown were safe and effective for children that an applicant has not brought to market within one year;
- that, for a product studied under this section, the labeling include study results (if they do or do not indicate safety and effectiveness, or if they are inconclusive) and the Secretary's determination;
- dissemination of labeling change information to health care providers; and
- reporting on the review of all adverse event reports and recommendations to the Secretary on actions in response.

Extended marketing exclusivity may be an attractive incentive to a manufacturer with a product that is being sold under patent or other types of exclusivity protections.[19] It is not, however, relevant in two cases: (1) when products are no longer covered by patent or other marketing exclusivity agreements and (2) when a patent-holding manufacturer declines to conduct the FDA-requested study and, therefore, the exclusivity.

FDA-NIH Collaboration
To encourage pediatric research that extends beyond FDA's authority to influence manufacturers' research plans, BPCA includes provisions to encourage pediatric research in products that involve the National Institutes of Health (NIH).

Off-Patent Products
BPCA 2002 addressed the first group, which it described as "off-patent," by adding a new Section 409I (42 U.S.C. 284m) to the Public Health Service Act (PHSA). The new section established an off-patent research fund at NIH for these studies and authorized appropriations of $200 million for FY2002 and such sums as necessary for each of the five years until the provisions were set to sunset on October 1, 2007. Congress repeated the authorization of appropriations in the 2007 legislation.

BPCA 2002 originally required the Secretary, through the NIH director and in consultation with the FDA commissioner and pediatric research experts, to list approved drugs for which pediatric studies were needed and to assess their safety and effectiveness. The 2007 reauthorization changed the specifications from an annual list of approved *drugs* to a list, revised every three years, of priority *study needs in pediatric therapeutics*, including drugs or indications. The Secretary is to determine (in consultation with the internal committee) whether a continuing need for pediatric studies exists. If so, the Secretary must refer those drugs for inclusion on the list. When the Secretary determines that drugs without pediatric studies require pediatric information, the Secretary must determine whether funds are available through the Foundation for the NIH (FNIH). If yes, the law requires the Secretary to issue a grant to conduct such studies. If no, it requires the Secretary to refer the drug for inclusion on the list established under PHSA Section 409I.

Manufacturer-Declined Studies

For on-patent drugs whose manufacturers declined FDA's written requests for studies, BPCA 2002 amended the FFDCA Section 505A to allow their referral by FDA to FNIH for pediatric studies, creating a second avenue of FDA-NIH collaboration.

The law requires the Secretary, after deciding that an on-patent drug requires pediatric study, to determine whether FNIH has sufficient money to fund a grant or contract for such studies. If it does, the Secretary must refer that study to FNIH and FNIH must fund it. If FNIH has insufficient funds, the Secretary may require the manufacturer to conduct a pediatric assessment under PREA (described in the Pediatric Research Equity Act section). If the Secretary does not require the study, the Secretary must notify the public of that decision and the reasons for it.

Other Provisions

BPCA 2002 also established an FDA Office of Pediatric Therapeutics, defined pediatric age groups to include neonates, and gave priority status to pediatric supplemental applications. BPCA 2007 includes requirements for the Secretary. It expanded the Secretary's authority and, in some cases, requires action. For example, the Secretary must publish within 30 days any determination regarding market exclusivity and must include a copy of the written request that specified what studies were necessary. The Secretary must also publicly identify any drug with a developed pediatric formulation that studies have demonstrated to be safe and effective for children if its manufacturer has not introduced the pediatric formulation onto the market within one year.

BPCA 2002 also required two outside reports. First, it required a report from the Comptroller General, in consultation with the HHS Secretary, on the effectiveness of the pediatric exclusivity program "in ensuring that medicines used by children are tested and properly labeled." By law, the report was to cover specified items such as the extent of testing, exclusivity determinations, labeling changes, and the economic impact of the program. GAO released its report in March 2007.[20] BPCA 2007 requires another report that GAO released in May 2011.[21]

Second, BPCA 2002 directed the HHS Secretary to contract with the Institute of Medicine (IOM) for a review of regulations, federally prepared or supported reports, and federally supported evidence-based research, all relating to research involving children.[22] The IOM report to Congress was to include recommendations on best practices relating to research involving children. IOM released its report in 2004. BPCA 2007 requires another IOM report.[23]

Pediatric Research Equity Act

After passing BPCA, Congress acted to provide statutory authority for actions FDA had been trying to achieve through regulation. (**Appendix B** provides a brief history of those attempts.) The goal was to have pediatric-appropriate labeling for all FDA-approved drug products. The Pediatric Research Equity Act of 2003 (PREA, P.L. 108-155) added to the FFDCA a new Section 505B (21 U.S.C. 355c): Research into Pediatric Uses for Drugs and Biological Products.[24] It includes requirements for both new applications and products already on the market.

LEGISLATIVE HISTORY OF PREA

Congress enacted the current PREA provisions in two separate pieces of legislation:

- the Pediatric Research Equity Act of 2003, essentially codifying a rule FDA promulgated in 1997; and
- the Pediatric Research Equity Act of 2007, enacted in the FDA Amendments Act.

See **Appendix B** for a discussion of the chronological development of BPCA and PREA.

New Applications

According to PREA, a manufacturer must submit a pediatric assessment[25] whenever it submits an application to market a new active ingredient, new indication, new dosage form, new dosing regimen, or new route of administration. Congress mandated that the submission be adequate to assess the safety and effectiveness of the product for the claimed indications in all relevant pediatric subpopulations, and that it support dosing and administration for each pediatric subpopulation for which the product is safe and effective. If the disease course and drug effects were sufficiently similar for adults and children, the HHS Secretary is authorized to allow extrapolation from adult study data as evidence of pediatric effectiveness. The manufacturer must document the data used to support such extrapolation, typically supplementing the evidence with other data from children, such as pharmacokinetic studies.[26]

The law specifies situations in which the Secretary might defer or waive the pediatric assessment requirement. For a deferral, an applicant must include a timeline for completion of studies. The Secretary must review each approved deferral annually, and applicants must submit documentation of study progress. All information from that review must promptly be made available to the public. In other situations, a waiver may be granted; for example, when the Secretary believes that doctors already know that a drug should never be used by children. In those cases, the law directs that the product's labeling include any waiver based on evidence that pediatric use would be unsafe or ineffective. If the Secretary waives the requirement to develop a pediatric formulation, the manufacturer must submit documentation detailing why a pediatric formulation could not be developed. The Secretary must promptly make available to the public all material submitted for granted waivers.

Products on the Market

PREA authorizes the Secretary to require the manufacturer of an approved drug or licensed biologic to submit a pediatric assessment. PREA 2002 and 2007 described the circumstances somewhat differently. The original provision applied to a drug used to treat a substantial number of pediatric patients for the labeled indications, and for which the *absence* of adequate labeling could pose *significant risks* to pediatric patients. PREA 2007, however, amended the provision so the Secretary could require a pediatric assessment of a drug for which the *presence* of adequate pediatric labeling "could confer a *benefit* on pediatric patients." PREA also applies when a drug might offer a meaningful therapeutic benefit over existing therapies for pediatric patients for one or more of the claimed indications.

Such situations could arise when the Secretary finds that a marketed product is being used by pediatric patients for indications labeled for adults, or that the product might provide children a meaningful therapeutic benefit over the available alternatives. The Secretary could require an assessment only after issuing a written request under FFDCA Section 505A (BPCA, pediatric exclusivity) or PHSA Section 409I (NIH funding mechanisms). Further, the manufacturer must not have agreed to conduct the assessment, and the Secretary had to have stated that the NIH funding programs either did or did not have enough funds to conduct that study.

If the manufacturer does not comply with the Secretary's request, the Secretary may consider the product misbranded. Because Congress wanted to protect adult access to a product under these circumstances, the law sets limits on FDA's enforcement options, precluding, for example, the withdrawal of approval or license to market.

Other Provisions

Under PREA, the Secretary must

- establish an internal committee, composed of FDA employees with specified expertise, to participate in the review of pediatric plans and assessments, deferrals, and waivers;
- track assessments and labeling changes and make that information publicly accessible; and
- establish a dispute resolution procedure, which would allow the commissioner, after specified steps, to deem a drug to be misbranded if a manufacturer refused to make a requested labeling change. The law includes review and reporting requirements for adverse events, and requires reports from both the IOM and the GAO.

Seeing PREA and BPCA as complementary approaches to the same goal, Congress, in 2003 and again in 2007, linked PREA to BPCA (a discussion of this linkage appears later in the "Issues for Reauthorization of BPCA and PREA" section). Therefore, rather than specify a sunset date, Congress authorized PREA to continue only as long as BPCA was in effect.

ISSUES FOR REAUTHORIZATION OF BPCA AND PREA

BPCA sunsets on October 1, 2012, and current law authorizes PREA only as long as BPCA is in effect. As Congress considers a 2012 reauthorization, issues may emerge that were contentious in the 2007 reauthorization discussions. Those include the relationship between the two laws, cost, measuring the impact of the programs, labeling, and enforcement. This section reviews each.

Relationship between BPCA and PREA

Although BPCA and PREA were developed separately, they are usually discussed—by policy analysts in FDA, Congress, and other interested organizations—in tandem. Their 2007 reauthorizations were paired in committee hearings and legislative vehicle (FDAAA) and Congress will likely consider them together in discussions of their 2012 reauthorizations. Now that BPCA and PREA have each been in effect for about a decade, it may be time to consider the rationale—whether planned or coincident—for two distinct approaches to encouraging pediatric drug research and product labeling.

Examining the Need for Pediatric Market Exclusivity

BPCA rewards pharmaceutical companies with extended market exclusivity for conducting studies on drugs for pediatric populations. In contrast, PREA requires pediatric studies. Legal analysts and some Members of Congress have speculated on this "carrot and stick" approach: Why Congress rewards the drug industry for something it requires the industry to do.

After reviewing the history of pediatric exclusivity when Congress was considering reauthorizing the FDAMA exclusivity provisions, one legal analyst wrote, in 2003:

> If Congress had codified the FDA's power to require testing in all new and already marketed drugs, the notion of an incentive or reward for testing would appear ludicrous.[27]

In fact, Congress did exactly that: provided an incentive for something that is already a requirement. During the debate on PREA in 2003, Members of the Senate differed on this issue. In the Committee on Health, Education, Labor, and Pensions' report, Chair Judd Gregg [28] wrote, "The Pediatric Rule[29] was intended to work as a ... backstop to ... pediatric exclusivity." Disagreeing, Senator Clinton and others wrote in the report's "Additional Views" section:

> Neither the intent conveyed by FDA nor FDA's implementation of the [Pediatric] [R]ule supports the report's contention that the rule was intended to work as a "backstop" to pediatric exclusivity or to be employed only to fill the gaps in coverage left by the exclusivity.

Three years later, in its draft guidance on "How to Comply with the Pediatric Research Equity Act," FDA wrote that "[t]he Pediatric Rule was designed to work in conjunction with the pediatric exclusivity provisions of section 505A of the Act."[30] However, development of the Pediatric Rule pre-dated development of the exclusivity provisions.

The unclear relationship between voluntary studies for marketing exclusivity in BPCA and mandatory studies in PREA remained, continued by FDAAA 2007. At some point Congress may want to resolve this apparent paradox.

If, however, Congress were to consider eliminating pediatric market exclusivity or to somehow combine BPCA and PREA provisions, it might need to realign what the provisions cover. A recent FDA committee report describes one such difference.[31] It noted that, because PREA "requires studies only in the specific indication or indications" addressed in the new drug application (NDA),[32] PREA assessments would not include potential uses of the drug that would be unique to a pediatric population and therefore not be noted as an adult indication. If, however, the manufacturer sought pediatric market exclusivity for that drug, the studies required under BPCA would cover all uses of the active drug component.

Examining the Need for Permanent PREA Authorization

Not every law contains a sunset provision. BPCA does, and, although Congress did not use the term, it structured PREA 2003 to cease if and when BPCA did, reflecting the majority approach discussed regarding "Relationship Between BPCA and PREA" above—that these are coordinated programs. Therefore, both BPCA and PREA are now set to end on October 1, 2012. By including an end date or another indication of a predetermined termination date, Congress provides "an 'action-forcing' mechanism, carrying the ultimate threat of termination, and a framework ... for the systematic review and evaluation of past performance."[33]

The sunset provision for BPCA's exclusivity incentive to manufacturers has not yet engendered congressional debate. However, during PREA consideration in 2003, some Members had objected, unsuccessfully, to linking PREA's safety and effectiveness assessment and resulting pediatric labeling to the BPCA sunset. By the committee markups of PREA in 2007, some Members advocated making the mandatory pediatric assessments permanent. If Congress intended the PREA sunset to trigger regular evaluation of the law's usefulness, other legislative approaches may achieve that result more directly, such as by requiring periodic evaluations.

If, however, the intent was to test the idea of requiring pediatric assessments, the years between PREA 2003 and consideration of PREA in 2007 had provided four years of evidence. The House-passed bill for PREA 2007 would have eliminated PREA's link to the BPCA sunset provision; the Senate-passed bill continued it.[34] The enacted bill included the linkage written in the 2003 legislation. As it approaches the 2012 reauthorization of these pediatric research provisions and with another five years of evidence, Congress may wish to evaluate the usefulness and effect of that link before it decides whether to continue it.

Costs and Benefits of Pediatric Marketing Exclusivity

In assessing the value of BPCA's offering of pediatric market exclusivity, it may be useful to identify the intended and unintended effects—both positive and negative—of its implementation. When FDA grants a manufacturer a six-month exclusivity, who might benefit and who might be harmed? Congress could consider the cost implications as it sets policy in the reauthorization.[35]

The manufacturer. The manufacturer holding pediatric exclusivity incurs the research and development expenses related to the FDA-requested pediatric studies. It then enjoys six months of sales without a competitor product and a potentially lucrative head start on future sales.

Some researchers have examined the *financial* costs and benefits faced by manufacturers that receive pediatric exclusivity. One 2007 study[36] calculated the net economic benefit (costs minus benefits, after estimating and adjusting for other factors) to a manufacturer that, in 2002-2004, responded to an FDA request for pediatric studies and received pediatric exclusivity. The median net economic benefit of six-month exclusivity was $134.3 million. The study found a large range, from a net loss of $9 million to a net benefit of over half a billion dollars.[37]

Other manufacturers. Manufacturers that do not hold the exclusivity must wait six months, during which time they cannot launch competing products. After that, however, they may be able to market generic versions of a drug that has been assessed for pediatric use and has had six months' experience in the public's awareness.

Government. Nonfinancial benefits to government include its progress in protecting children's health. Financial costs to the government include administrative and regulatory expenses. Because the government also pays for drugs, both directly and indirectly, it must pay the higher price that exclusivity allows by deferring the availability of lower-priced generics for six months.[38] The improved pediatric information, however, may yield future financial savings by avoiding ineffective and unsafe uses.

Private insurers. Private payers also face similar financial costs and benefits as public payers, without the regulatory costs of administering the program.

Children and their families. If the six-month exclusivity incentives effectively encourage manufacturers to study their drugs in children, some children may incur risks as study subjects; conversely, they and others might benefit from more appropriate use of drugs, including accurate dosing.

Labeling

Pediatric studies can produce valuable information about safety, effectiveness, dosing, and side effects when a child takes a medication. Such information benefits children only when it reaches clinicians and others who care for children (including parents). BPCA 2002, PREA 2003, and their 2007 reauthorizations, therefore, included labeling provisions to make the information available. As Congress drafts language to continue BPCA and PREA, it could address whether FDA has adequate tools with which to assess, encourage, require, and enforce the development and dissemination of the information clinicians could use to reach better treatment decisions. Before examining some specific questions for congressional consideration, this report reviews the current requirements for pediatric labeling.

Current Pediatric Labeling Requirements

FDA now requires, by law, pediatric usage information labeling in the following three sets of circumstances:

1. the manufacturer has successfully applied (via an original new drug application [NDA] or a supplement) for approval to list a pediatric indication;[39]
2. the manufacturer has received pediatric exclusivity after conducting appropriate studies;[40] or
3. the manufacturer has submitted the safety and effectiveness findings from pediatric assessments required under PREA (added by the 2007 reauthorization).

By regulation, FDA requires pediatric-specific labeling in the following circumstances:[41]

(B) If there is a specific pediatric indication different from those approved for adults that is supported by adequate and well-controlled studies in the pediatric population, …
(C) If there are specific statements on pediatric use of the drug for an indication also approved for adults that are based on adequate and well-controlled studies in the pediatric population, …
(D)(1) When a drug is approved for pediatric use based on adequate and well-controlled studies in adults with other information supporting pediatric use, …
(E) If the requirements for a finding of substantial evidence to support a pediatric indication or a pediatric use statement have not been met for a particular pediatric population, …
(F) If the requirements for a finding of substantial evidence to support a pediatric indication or a pediatric use statement have not been met for any pediatric population, …
(G) … FDA may permit use of an alternative statement if FDA determines that no statement described in those paragraphs is appropriate or relevant to the drug's labeling and that the alternative statement is accurate and appropriate.

(H) If the drug product contains one or more inactive ingredients that present an increased risk of toxic effects to neonates or other pediatric subgroups, ...

The PREA and BPCA reauthorizations in 2007 added the third set of circumstances of required pediatric labeling. When the Secretary determines that a pediatric assessment or study does or does not demonstrate that the subject drug is safe and effective in pediatric populations or subpopulations, the Secretary must order the label to include information about those results and a statement of the Secretary's determination. That is true even if the study results were inconclusive.

If studies suggest that safety, effectiveness, or dosage reactions vary by age, condition to be treated, or patient circumstances, then detailed information could be included in the labeling.

BPCA 2007 also strengthened the effect of labeling requirements by mandating the dissemination of certain safety and effectiveness information to health care providers and the public.

Although not included in the pediatric sections, another provision in FDAAA 2007 may yield benefits for pediatric labeling. Regarding television and radio direct-to-consumer (DTC) drug advertisements, the law required that major statements relating to side effects and contraindications be presented in a clear, conspicuous, and neutral manner. It further required that the Secretary establish standards for determining whether a major statement meets those criteria.[42] The fruits of such inquiry could be applied throughout FDA communication.

Finally, BPCA 2003 had required HHS to promulgate a rule within one year of enactment regarding the placement on all drug labels of a toll-free telephone number for reporting adverse events.[43] Because FDA had not yet finalized a proposed rule it had issued in 2004, BPCA 2007 required that it take effect on January 1, 2008.[44]

Questions for Congressional Consideration

Labeling is useful if its statements are clear and applicable to the decision at hand. The labeling must also, however, be available and read—at least by prescribing clinicians. While an improvement over no mention at all, a statement such as "effectiveness in pediatric patients has not been established" still deprives a clinician of available information. The statement does not distinguish among

- *studies in children found the drug to be ineffective;*
- *studies in children found the drug to be unsafe;*
- *studies in children were not conclusive regarding safety or effectiveness; and*
- *no studies had been conducted concerning pediatric use.*

With BPCA and PREA, Congress has acted to encourage more informative labeling and the research that would make that possible. Having observed a decade of experience with these requirements, Congress may want to ask follow-up questions to help determine whether the laws need amending. Have the dissemination provisions mandated by BPCA 2007 been adequate? Has FDA been able to enforce the labeling changes that the agency deems necessary based on results of pediatric studies under BPCA and PREA? Should Congress consider strengthening enforcement provisions in the reauthorization bill? Now that the law requires all labeling to require a toll-free number for reporting adverse events, might Congress want to explore how that is implemented and whether it has had any effect?

Measuring the Impact on Pediatric Drug Research

Have the pediatric research encouragement programs had an effect? Is more research done on pediatric safety and effectiveness? Is more detail on age-group pharmacodynamics and dosing added to labeling? In general, is more information available to clinicians that could help them make appropriate prescribing decisions?

BPCA and PREA have created a measurable change in the numbers of drugs with labeling that includes pediatric-specific information. Still, not all drugs used by children have labeling that addresses pediatric use. FDA approved more than 1,000 new drug and biologics license applications from the beginning of 2003 through 2009.[45] Yet, the PREA (and its predecessor Pediatric Rule) and BPCA statistics note 394 pediatric labeling changes since 1998.[46]

FDA, through BPCA, has granted pediatric exclusivity for pediatric studies for 178 drugs.[47] Those drugs make up 45% of the drugs for which FDA had sent written requests to manufacturers for pediatric studies. FDA did not grant exclusivity for 14 drugs for which manufacturers had submitted studies in response to requests, but manufacturers did not pursue exclusivity for most of the other drugs.

As described earlier, BPCA 2007 shifted the level at which NIH set pediatric research priorities. Rather than creating a drug-specific list, NIH creates a condition-specific list. Accordingly, NIH (coordinated by the Obstetric and Pediatric Pharmacology Branch of the National Institute of Child Health and Human Development [NICHD]) listed 34 "priority needs in pediatric therapeutics," basically medical conditions, and interventions for each. Of the 45 drugs mentioned, 5 were still covered by their manufacturers' patents. Also listed were a few non-drug interventions: drug delivery systems (for asthma, for nerve agent exposure), health literacy (for over-the-counter drug use), and devices used in dialysis (for chronic liver failure).[48] It may be interesting to see whether this shift in priorities from drugs to conditions affects the funding of specific research and ultimate availability of pediatric-specific drug labeling.

Since BPCA and PREA were reauthorized in FDAAA, several reports have examined how FDA has implemented their requirements. GAO and the FDA Pediatric Review Committee (PeRC) that FDAAA established have offered assessments and recommendations for improvement. Congress may be interested in exploring those findings and crafting those recommendations into possible amendments to current law.

In May 2011, GAO reported to Congress, as required by PREA 2007, a description of the effects of BPCA and PREA since their 2007 reauthorization.[49] Along with a description of the procedures required by the provisions, GAO notes an area in which FDA needs to improve data resources in order to better manage the programs. Although FDA can report the number of completed PREA assessments, it was unable to provide a count of applications subject to PREA. GAO points out that, without that information, it is difficult for FDA to manage its timetables and for others to assess PREA's effect. In describing concerns of stakeholders, GAO mentions "confusion about how to comply with PREA and BPCA due to a lack of current guidance from FDA" and difficulties in coordinating the differing content and timetables of U.S. and European Union pediatric study requirements.

As required by PREA 2007, FDA created an internal expert committee—the Pediatric Review Committee (PeRC)—that, among other things, conducted a retrospective review of assessments, waivers, and deferrals under PREA through September 2007.[50] The required PeRC report found that, although the pediatric assessments were "generally of good scientific quality," if FDA provided more detailed advice on what it wanted, the assessments could be more consistent and useful. In a related observation, PeRC noted that "where there is evidence of specific discussion and documentation of the studies need to fulfill the PREA requirements ..., the PREA assessments generally were of higher quality."

Inconsistency in decisions about waivers and deferrals were seen in the earlier years of PREA and the report noted that with the PREA 2007-required PeRC, a higher level of pediatric drug development expertise was now available to support all 17 review divisions, some of which had no pediatricians on staff.

PeRC recommended that plans for and conduct of pediatric studies should begin early in the process of NDA development. This would be useful, in particular, to "correct problems in consistency between pediatric assessments in response to a Written Request [for BPCA] and those only in response to the PREA requirement." In keeping with its concern over varied scope and quality of research designs, PeRC recommended that (1) FDA review divisions discuss plans in detail approaching what they would cover in a BPCA Written Request to "be better able to assess the scope of studies need to provide adequate data for dosing, safety, and efficacy for use in the appropriate pediatric populations;" and (2) FDA provide more extensive descriptions of PREA postmarketing study requirements in its approval letters.

PeRC recommended that when assessments come after an application is approved, FDA should ask the manufacturer to submit a labeling supplement as required by PREA 2007. Furthermore, finding that "[r]esults from pediatric assessments were not consistently incorporated into labeling," PeRC suggested that "[c]onsistency in placement and language may increase the ability of clinicians and patients/guardians to find information in the label" and recommended that FDA issue a pediatric labeling guidance.

Enforcement

FDA's postmarket authority regarding pediatric drug use labeling has been limited. Congress had given FDA the authority to use its most powerful enforcement tool—deeming a product to be "misbranded" and thereby being able to pull it from the market—but has not given the agency authority to require less drastic actions, such as labeling changes. Of interest to Congress may be whether the current authority is appropriate and sufficient to ensure safety and, therefore, whether FDA should have a wider range of options.

Pulling from the market a drug that many consumers rely on could, according to some health care analysts, do more harm than good. In its report accompanying its PREA 2003 bill, the Senate committee noted its intent that the misbranding authority regarding pediatric use labeling not be the basis for criminal proceedings or withdrawal of approval, and only rarely result in seizure of the offending product.[51] The 2007 reauthorization continued this limitation on misbranding authority.

The FDAAA, which encompassed BPCA 2007 and PREA 2007, included a provision outside its pediatric-specific sections to create a new enforcement authority for FDA: civil monetary penalties. Framed in the context of giving FDA tools to create meaningful incentives for manufacturer compliance with a range of postmarket safety activities, the provision listed labeling within its scope. In 2007 Senate and House committee discussions of what maximum penalties to allow, proposed one-time penalties were as low as $15,000 and proposed upper levels ranged up to $50 million. The enacted bill (FDAAA) states that an applicant violating certain requirements regarding postmarket safety, studies or clinical trials, or *labeling* is subject to a civil monetary penalty of not more than $250,000 per violation, and not to exceed $1 million for all such violations adjudicated in a single proceeding. If a violation continues after the Secretary provides notice of such violation to the applicant, the Secretary may impose a civil penalty of $250,000 for the first 30 days, doubling for every subsequent 30-day period, up to $1 million for one 30-day period, and up to $10 million for all such violations adjudicated in a single proceeding. The Secretary must, in determining the amount of civil penalty, consider whether the manufacturer is attempting to correct the violation.

What options should FDA have if a manufacturer that has already received the six-month pediatric exclusivity then refuses or delays making an appropriate labeling change? For studies that result in labeling changes, when should FDA make study results available to the public? In considering whether to strengthen FDA's enforcement authority within the context of pediatric research and labeling, Congress can address manufacturers' actions at many points in the regulatory process, if and when, for example, FDA notes a manufacturer's reluctance to accept the agency's requested study scope, design, and timetable; that a study's completion is clearly lagging or overdue; that a manufacturer does not complete such a study; or does not release its results to FDA, peer-reviewed publications, or the public; or that procedures to incorporate pediatric study results into a drug's labeling have not proceeded appropriately.

CONCLUDING COMMENTS

Congress has repeatedly acted to encourage research into the unique effects of FDA-regulated drugs on children—with both "carrots" of financial incentive and "sticks" of required action. It has also required that drug labeling reflect the findings of pediatric research, whether positive, negative, or inconclusive. And, most recently, it has given FDA broader authority to enforce these requirements.

With each step of legislative and regulatory action over the years, Congress and FDA have tried to balance often conflicting goals:

- drug development to address needs unique to children;
- tools to encourage drug manufacturers to test drugs for use in children, despite the expense, opportunity costs, and liability risk;
- protection of children as subjects of clinical research;
- public access to up-to-date and unbiased information on drug safety and effectiveness; and
- prioritizing agency activities in light of available resources.

Concerns remain, though, about many of the issues discussed during the 2007 reauthorizations— as well as issues presented in the last section of this report. Such issues may surface when reauthorizations are due in 2012 or in the broader context of congressional interest in drug safety and effectiveness.

APPENDIX A. ACRONYMS

BLA	Biologics License Application
BPCA	Best Pharmaceuticals for Children Act
C.F.R.	Code of Federal Regulations
DTC	direct-to-consumer (as in DTC advertising)
FDA	Food and Drug Administration
FDAAA	FDA Amendments Act of 2007
FDAMA	FDA Modernization Act
FFDCA	Federal Food, Drug, and Cosmetic Act
FNIH	Foundation for the National Institutes of Health
GAO	Government Accountability Office

HHS	Department of Health and Human Services
IOM	Institute of Medicine
NDA	New Drug Application
NICHD	National Institute of Child Health and Human Development
NIH	National Institutes of Health
PeRC	Pediatric Review Committee
PHSA	Public Health Service Act
PREA	Pediatric Research Equity Act
U.S.C.	United States Code

APPENDIX B. CURRENT LAW EVOLVED FROM EARLIER ATTEMPTS

Before BPCA 2002 and PREA 2003, FDA attempted to spur pediatric drug research through administrative action. **Table B-1** shows the administrative and statutory efforts to encourage pediatric drug research. The following discussion highlights selected FDA-specific rules and statutes that relate to discussions in this report.

Rule on Drug Labeling: 1979

In a 1979 rule on drug labeling (21 C.F.R. Part 201), FDA established a "Pediatric use" subsection.[52] The rule required that labeling include pediatric dosage information for a drug with a specific pediatric indication (approved use of the drug). It also required that statements regarding pediatric use for indications approved for adults be based on "substantial evidence derived from adequate and well-controlled studies" or that the labeling include the statement, "Safety and effectiveness in children have not been established."[53]

Despite the 1979 rule, most prescription drug labels continued to lack adequate pediatric use information. The requirement for adequate and well-controlled studies deterred many manufacturers who, apparently, did not understand that the rule included a waiver option.[54] FDA, therefore, issued another rule in 1994.

Table B-1. Administrative and Statutory Efforts to Encourage Pediatric Drug Research

Year	Action
1977	FDA pediatric guidance on "General Considerations for the Clinical Evaluation of Drugs in Infants and Children"[a]
1979[b]	FDA rule on *Pediatric Use* subsection of product package insert: *Precautions* section [21 C.F.R. 201.57] (in 44 Fed. Reg. 37434)
1994[b]	FDA rule revised
1996	FDA guidance on "Content and Format of Pediatric Use Section"[c]
1997[b]	Food and Drug Administration Modernization Act (FDAMA, P.L. 105-115), included the Better Pharmaceuticals for Children Act
1998[b]	FDA Pediatric Rule finalized (effective 1999; invalidated by a federal court in 2002)
2001	Adaptation of HHS Subpart D (pediatric) regulations [45 C.F.R. 46 Subpart D] to FDA-regulated research [21 C.F.R. 50 Subpart D]
2002	Best Pharmaceuticals for Children Act (BPCA, P.L. 107-109)
2003	Pediatric Research Equity Act (PREA, P.L. 108-155)
2007	FDA Amendments Act of 2007 (FDAAA, P.L. 110-85) reauthorized BPCA and PREA and enacted the Pediatric Medical Device Safety and Improvement Act

Source: CRS adapted and expanded material from Steven Hirschfeld, Division of Oncology Drug Products & Division of Pediatric Drug Development, Center for Drug Evaluation and Research (CDER), FDA, "History of Pediatric Labeling," presentation to the Pediatric Oncology Subcommittee of the Oncologic Drugs Advisory Committee, March 4, 2003, at http://www.fda.gov/?ohrms/?dockets/?ac/?03/?slides/?3927S1_01_Hirshfeld%20.ppt.

a. FDA, "Guidance for Industry: General Considerations for the Clinical Evaluation of Drugs in Infants and Children," September 2007, http://www.fda.gov/downloads/Drugs/GuidanceComplianceRegulatory Information/Guidances/ucm071687.pdf.

b. Discussed in Appendix text.

c. FDA, "Guidance for Industry: The Content and Format for Pediatric Use Supplements," May 1996, http://www.fda.gov/downloads/Drugs/Guidance ComplianceRegulatoryInformation/Guidances/ucm071957.pdf.

Revised Rule: 1994

The revised rule attempted to make clear that the "adequate and well-controlled studies" language did not require that manufacturers conduct clinical trials in children. The new rule described how FDA would determine whether the evidence was substantial and adequate. If, for example, clinicians would use the drug to treat a different condition in children than its FDA-approved use in adults, FDA would require trials in children. However, if the drug would be used in children for the same condition for which FDA had approved its use in adults, the labeling statement regarding effectiveness could be based on adult trials alone. In such instances, FDA might also require pediatric study-based data on pharmacokinetics or relevant safety measures. The 1994 rule continued the 1979 requirement that manufacturers include statements regarding uses for which there was no substantial evidence of safety and effectiveness. It added a requirement that labels include information about known specific hazards from the active or inactive ingredients.[55]

Food and Drug Administration Modernization Act of 1997

Three years later, Congress provided another approach to increasing pediatric labeling. FDAMA (P.L. 105-115), incorporating the provisions introduced as the Better Pharmaceuticals for Children Act, created a Section 505A (21 U.S.C. 355a) in the FFDCA: Pediatric Studies of Drugs. It provided drug manufacturers with an incentive to conduct pediatric use studies on their patented products. If a manufacturer completed a pediatric study according to FDA's written request, which included design, size, and other specifications, FDA would extend its market exclusivity for that product for six months.[56] The law required that the Secretary publish an annual list of FDA-approved drugs for which additional pediatric information might produce health benefits. FDAMA also required that the Secretary prepare a report examining whether the new law enhanced pediatric use information, whether the incentive was adequate, and what the program's economic impact was on taxpayers and consumers.

Pediatric Rule: Proposed 1997, Finalized 1998, Effective 1999-2002

Also in 1997, FDA issued a proposed regulation that came to be called the Pediatric Rule.[57] The Pediatric Rule mandated that manufacturers submit pediatric testing data at the time of all new drug applications to FDA. The rule went into effect in 1999, prompting a lawsuit against FDA by the Competitive

Enterprise Institute and the Association of American Physicians and Surgeons. The plaintiffs claimed that the agency was acting outside its authority in considering off-label uses of approved drugs. In October 2002, a federal court declared the Pediatric Rule invalid, noting that its finding related not to the rule's policy value but to FDA's statutory authority in promulgating it:

> The Pediatric Rule may well be a better policy tool than the one enacted by Congress (which encourages testing for pediatric use, but does not require it).... It might reflect the most thoughtful, reasoned, balanced solution to a vexing public health problem. The issue here is not the Rule's wisdom.... The issue is the Rule's statutory authority, and it is this that the court finds wanting.[58]

End Notes

[1] Estimates vary between 65%-85%, perhaps because analysts use different denominators (e.g., all drugs, or all drugs used by children). See, for example, Statement of Rear Admiral Sandra Lynn Kweder, M.D., Deputy Director, Office of New Drugs, Center for Drug Evaluation and Research, "Programs Affecting Safety and Innovation in Pediatric Therapies," before the Subcommittee on Health, House Committee on Energy and Commerce, May 22, 2007,http://www.fda.gov/NewsEvents/Testimony/ucm153848.htm.

[2] Best Pharmaceuticals for Children Act (BPCA) of 2002, P.L. 107-109. Pediatric Research Equity Act (PREA) of 2003, P.L. 108-155. For a list of acronyms used in this report, see **Appendix A**.

[3] In FDAAA, Congress also created a program to address medical devices used in children—the Pediatric Medical Device Safety and Improvement Act (PMDSIA) of 2007. See CRS Report RL32826, *The Medical Device Approval Process and Related Legislative Issues*, by Erin D. Williams.

[4] CRS Report RL34465, *FDA Amendments Act of 2007 (P.L. 110-85)*, by Erin D. Williams and Susan Thaul, presents detailed descriptions of these and other FDAAA provisions.

[5] FDA describes "indication" as a "[d]escription of use of drug in the treatment, prevention or diagnosis of a recognized disease or condition" (FDA, "Drug Development and Review Definitions," http://www.fda.gov/Drugs/DevelopmentApprovalProcess/HowDrugsareDevelopedandAppr oved/ApprovalApplications/InvestigationalNewDrugINDApplication/ucm176522.htm).

[6] For descriptions and discussions of the FDA procedure for approving new drugs, see CRS Report R41983, *How FDA Approves Drugs and Regulates Their Safety and Effectiveness*, by Susan Thaul, and FDA, "Development & Approval Process (Drugs)," http://www.fda. gov/Drugs/DevelopmentApprovalProcess/default.htm (see links).

[7] Federal Food, Drug, and Cosmetic Act (FFDCA), 21 U.S.C. §301 et seq.

[8] The FFDCA does not give FDA authority to regulate the practice of medicine; that responsibility rests with the states and medical professional associations.

[9] David A. Williams, Haiming Xu, and Jose A. Cancelas, "Children are not little adults: just ask their hematopoietic stem cells," *J Clin Invest.*, vol. 116, no. 10, October 2, 2006, pp. 2593-2596; and Stephen Ashwal (Editor), *The Founders of Child Neurology* (San Francisco: Norman Publishing, 1990).

[10] William Rodriguez, Office of New Drugs, FDA, "What We Learned from the Study of Drugs Under the Pediatric Initiatives," June 2006 presentation to the Institute of Medicine.

[11] Examples taken from a presentation by Dianne Murphy, Director, Office of Pediatric Therapeutics, Office of the Commissioner, FDA, "Impact of Pediatric Legislative Initiatives: USA," January 26, 2005, presentation to the European Forum for Good Clinical Practice; and Rodriguez, June 2006. Other sources include W. Rodriguez, A. Selen, D. Avant, C. Chaurasia, T. Crescenzi, G. Gieser, J. Di Giacinto, S.M. Huang, P. Lee, L. Mathis, D. Murphy, S. Murphy, R. Roberts, H.C. Sachs, S. Suarez, V. Tandon, and R.S. Uppoor, "Improving pediatric dosing through pediatric initiatives: what we have learned," *Pediatrics*, vol. 121, no. 3 (March 2008), pp. 530-539.

[12] See, for example, Statement of Rear Admiral Sandra Lynn Kweder, M.D., Deputy Director, Office of New Drugs, Center for Drug Evaluation and Research, "Programs Affecting Safety and Innovation in Pediatric Therapies," before the Subcommittee on Health, House Committee on Energy and Commerce, May 22, 2007, http://www.fda.gov/NewsEvents/ Testimony/ucm153848.htm.

[13] HHS regulations are in 45 C.F.R. 46 Subpart D. FDA regulations are in 21 C.F.R. 50 Subpart D. Protection of children in research is discussed in CRS Report RL32909, *Federal Protection for Human Research Subjects: An Analysis of the Common Rule and Its Interactions with FDA Regulations and the HIPAA Privacy Rule*, by Erin D. Williams. See, also, Institute of Medicine, *The Ethical Conduct of Clinical Research Involving Children*, Washington, D.C.: National Academies Press, 2004.

[14] CRS Report RL34465, *FDA Amendments Act of 2007 (P.L. 110-85)*, by Erin D. Williams and Susan Thaul, presents detailed tables comparing FDAAA 2007 with BPCA 2002 and PREA 2003, showing both changed and unchanged provisions.

[15] See, for example, FDA, "Should Your Child Be in a Clinical Trial?," January 13, 2010, http:// www.fda.gov/ForConsumers/ConsumerUpdates/ucm048699.htm.

[16] The FFDCA authorizes marketing exclusivity in specified circumstances for pediatric studies, orphan drugs, new chemicals, patent challenges (FDA, "Frequently Asked Questions on Patents and Exclusivity," http://www.fda.gov/Drugs/DevelopmentApprovalProcess/ ucm079031.htm).

[17] The laws refer to the *sponsor* of an application or the *holder* of an approved application. Because that entity is usually the product's manufacturer, this report uses the term *manufacturer* throughout.

[18] Authority under BPCA 2007 will sunset on October 1, 2012.

[19] The FFDCA authorizes marketing exclusivity in specified circumstances for pediatric studies, orphan drugs, new chemicals, patent challenges (FDA, "Frequently Asked Questions on Patents and Exclusivity," http://www.fda.gov/Drugs/DevelopmentApprovalProcess/ ucm079031.htm).

[20] In March 2007, the Government Accountability Office (GAO) issued a report that the BPCA legislation had required (GAO, *Pediatric Drug Research: Studies Conducted under Best Pharmaceuticals for Children Act*, Report to Congressional Committees, GAO-07-557, March 2007). Noting that most of the exclusivity-associated studies resulted in labeling changes, GAO calculated the time that elapsed before those changes were completed. The entire process— from initial data submission, through FDA review and frequent requests for additional data, to follow-up submissions and reviews—took an average of nine months. One-third of the drugs' labeling changing took less than three months, whereas the labeling change for one drug took almost three years. The GAO report identified three main categories of labeling change: to inform of ineffective drugs, dosing that was too high or too low, and newly identified adverse events. It juxtaposed those findings with the statement that children take many of these drugs for common, serious, or life-threatening conditions.

[21] BPCA 2007 (FDAAA) directed that GAO submit a report by January 1, 2011. GAO briefed the committees on its findings on December 15, 2010, and later submitted its report (GAO,

Pediatric Research: Products Studied under Two Related Laws, but Improved Tracking Needed by FDA, Report to Congressional Committees, GAO-11-457, May 2011).

[22] See Institute of Medicine (IOM), *Ethical Conduct of Clinical Research Involving Children*, Committee on Clinical Research Involving Children (Washington, DC: National Academies Press, 2004), done with funding from NIH and FDA.

[23] BPCA 2007 (FDAAA) directed that the Secretary enter a contract with IOM by September 27, 2010. IOM has formed an ad hoc committee to consider "Pediatric Studies Conducted under BPCA and PREA"; it anticipates releasing a final report by February 2012.

[24] Unlike BPCA, which applied only to drugs, PREA applied both to drugs regulated under the FFDCA and to biological products (e.g., vaccines) regulated under the PHSA. In 2010, the Patient Protection and Affordable Care Act (ACA, P.L. 111-148) amended BPCA to add a pediatric market exclusivity provision for biological products.

[25] FFDCA '505B(a)(2)(A) describes the assessment as follows: "The assessments referred to in paragraph (1) shall contain data, gathered using appropriate formulations for each age group for which the assessment is required, that are adequate—(i) to assess the safety and effectiveness of the drug or the biological product for the claimed indications in all relevant pediatric subpopulations; and (ii) to support dosing and administration for each pediatric subpopulation for which the drug or the biological product is safe and effective."

[26] PREA 2007 authorized the Secretary to calculate pediatric effectiveness by extrapolating from adult data in certain circumstances. FDA cautions that "selection of an appropriate dose ... and the assessment of pediatric-specific safety should never be extrapolated" and that even efficacy extrapolation "requires an understanding of disease pathophysiology and the mechanism of therapeutic response" (Robert M. Nelson, Pediatric Ethicist, FDA Office of Pediatric Therapeutics, "21 C.F.R. 50, Subpart D: Additional Safeguards for Children in Clinical Investigations of FDA-Regulated Products," presentation to the Pediatric Ethics Subcommittee of the FDA Pediatric Advisory Committee, June 9, 2008, http://www.fda. gov/ohrms/dockets/ac/08/slides/2008-4399s1-13%20%28Nelson%20Presentation%29.pdf).

[27] Lauren Hammer Breslow, "The Best Pharmaceuticals for Children Act of 2002: The Rise of the Voluntary Incentive Structure and Congressional Refusal to Require Pediatric Testing," *Harvard Journal on Legislation*, vol. 40, 2003, pp. 133-191.

[28] S.Rept. 108-84, to accompany S. 650, the Pediatric Research Equity Act of 2003, June 27, 2003.

[29] PREA effectively codified the FDA-promulgated Pediatric Rule; see **Appendix B** for additional detail.

[30] FDA "DRAFT Guidance for Industry: How to Comply with the Pediatric Research Equity Act," Center for Drug Evaluation and Research (CDER) and Center for Biologics Evaluation and Research (CBER), September 2005. http://www.fda.gov/downloads/Drugs/GuidanceComplianceRegulatoryInformation/Guidances/ucm079756.pdf.

[31] FDA Pediatric Review Committee (PeRC), "Retrospective Review of Information Submitted and Actions Taken in Response to PREA 2003," January 14, 2010, http://www.fda.gov/downloads/Drugs/DevelopmentApprovalProcess/DevelopmentResources/UCM197636.pdf.

[32] For a description of the drug approval process, see CRS Report R41983, *How FDA Approves Drugs and Regulates Their Safety and Effectiveness*, by Susan Thaul.

[33] CRS Report RS21210, *Sunset Review: A Brief Introduction*, by Virginia A. McMurtry.

[34] Not all Senate committee members agreed. See, for example, Senator Clinton's comments at the Senate Committee on Health, Education, Labor, and Pensions hearing, "Ensuring Safe Medicines and Medical Devices for Children," March 27, 2007, at http://www.cq.com/?display.do?dockey=/?cqonline/?prod/?data/?docs/?html/?transcripts/?congressional/?110/?congressionaltranscripts110-000002481833.html@committees&metapub=CQ-CONGTRANSCRIPTS&searchIndex=0&seqNum=13; and S.Rept. 108-84, Additional Views.

[35] For example, although the BPCA reauthorization in 2007 continued the six-month exclusivity, the Senate bills under consideration at the time (S. 1082 and S. 1156 in the 110th Congress)

would have limited the period of exclusivity for a drug to three months if its manufacturer/sponsor had more than $1 billion in annual gross U.S. sales for all its products with the same active ingredient. In future years, Congress might reexamine whether such limits are in the public interest.

[36] Jennifer S. Li, Eric L. Eisenstein, Henry G. Grabowski, et al., "Economic Return of Clinical Trials Performed Under the Pediatric Exclusivity Program," *Journal of the American Medical Association*, vol. 297, no. 5, February 7, 2007, pp. 480-488.

[37] An indepth examination of the financial effects of pediatric exclusivity is beyond the scope of this report.

[38] For example, a University of Utah research group examined the effect of the six-month pediatric market exclusivity on costs incurred by the Utah Medicaid program for three classes of drugs. Their extrapolation of Utah's $2.2 million extra cost led to a national Medicaid estimate of $430 million for those three drug classes over an 18-month period. (Carrie McAdam-Marx, Megan L. Evans, Robert Ward, Benjamin Campbell, Diana Brixner, Joanne Lafleur, Richard E. Nelson, Patent Extension Policy for Paediatric Indications, *Applied Health Economics and Health Policy*, vol. 9, no. 3, May 2011, p. 171).

[39] In the first case, the labeling includes pediatric use information only if FDA approved the pediatric indication. If FDA turned down or the manufacturer withdrew a request for a pediatric indication, pediatric use information appears nowhere in the product's labeling. In addition, the fact that the manufacturer had made an unsuccessful attempt—and the research findings that blocked approval—would be neither noted in the label nor made public in other ways.

[40] When it comes to exclusivity, the labeling rules are different. If the studies required for exclusivity support pediatric use or specific limits to pediatric use (different dosing or subgroups), that information would go in the labeling. The labeling would also make clear if the studies did not find the drug to be effective in children or if FDA waived the requirement to study because children should not or would not be given the drug.

[41] Material is abstracted from 21 C.F.R. 201.57(c)(9)(iv).

[42] FDA, 21 C.F.R. Part 202 [Docket No. FDA–2009–N–0582] "Direct-to-Consumer Prescription Drug Advertisements; Presentation of the Major Statement in Television and Radio Advertisements in a Clear, Conspicuous, and Neutral Manner; Proposed rule," *Federal Register*, vol. 75, no. 59, March 29, 2010, pp. 15376-15387.

[43] FDA collects reports of adverse events from consumers, clinicians, and manufacturers. CRS Report R41983, *How FDA Approves Drugs and Regulates Their Safety and Effectiveness*, by Susan Thaul, describes FDA's authority and activities regarding adverse event report collection, review, analysis, and subsequent agency action.

[44] FDA issued the final rule on October 28, 2008. Its effective date is November 28, 2008, and its compliance date is July 1, 2009 (FDA [21 C.F.R. Parts 201, 208, and 209], "Toll-Free Number for Reporting Adverse Events on Labeling for Human Drug Products; Final rule," *Federal Register*, vol. 73, no. 209, October 28, 2008, pp. 63886-63897). BPCA 2007 limited the rule's application to exclude certain drugs whose packaging already includes a toll-free number for consumers to report complaints to their manufacturers or distributors.

[45] For more information, see FDA, "Drug and Biologic Approval Reports," http://www.fda.gov/ Drugs/DevelopmentApprovalProcess/HowDrugsareDevelopedandApproved/DrugandBiolo gicApprovalReports/default.htm.

[46] FDA, "Pediatric Labeling Changes through September 28, 2010," http://www.fda.gov/ downloads/ScienceResearch/SpecialTopics/PediatricTherapeuticsResearch/UCM221329.cs v.

[47] The count is based on BPCA statistics through 2010 (FDA, "Drugs to Which FDA has Granted Pediatric Exclusivity for Pediatric Studies under Section 505A of the Federal Food, Drug, and Cosmetic Act," http://www.fda.gov/Drugs/DevelopmentApprovalProcess/ DevelopmentResources/ucm0500005.htm).

[48] National Institute of Child Health and Human Development, "Priority List of Needs in Pediatric Therapeutics for 2008-2009 as of September 1, 2009," http://bpca.nichd.nih.gov/about/process/upload/2009-Summary-091509-1-rev.pdf. NIH also pursues pediatric drug research outside of its role in BPCA and PREA. For example, in August 2010, NICHD announced a request for grant applications (RFA) to address not yet understood molecular and other mechanisms of known side effects in children of atypical antipsychotics, cardiovascular drugs, highly active antiretroviral therapies, and depro-medroxyprogesterone acetate (NIH, "Molecular Mechanisms of Adverse Metabolic Drug Effects in Children and Adolescents(R01)," Request for Applications (RFA) Number: RFA-HD-10-010, http://grants.nih.gov/grants/guide/rfa-files/RFA-HD-10-010.html).

[49] GAO, *Pediatric Research: Products Studied under Two Related Laws, but Improved Tracking Needed by FDA*, Report to Congressional Committees, GAO-11-457, May 2011.

[50] FDA Pediatric Review Committee (PeRC), "Retrospective Review of Information Submitted and Actions Taken in Response to PREA 2003," January 14, 2010, http://www.fda.gov/downloads/Drugs/DevelopmentApprovalProcess/DevelopmentResources/UCM197636.pdf.

[51] S.Rept. 108-84.

[52] Originally at 21 C.F.R. 201.57(f)(9), this material is now at 21 C.F.R. 201.57(c)(9)(iv).

[53] FDA, "Labeling and Prescription Drug Advertising; Content and Format for Labeling for Human Prescription Drugs; Final rule," *Federal Register*, vol. 44, no. 124, June 26, 1979, pp. 37434-37467.

[54] FDA would waive the required pediatric assessment for a drug that "does not represent a meaningful therapeutic benefit over existing treatments for pediatric patients and is not likely to be used in a substantial number of pediatric patients;" or for which "necessary studies are impossible or highly impractical because the number of patients is so small or geographically dispersed; or "there is evidence strongly suggesting that the drug product would be ineffective or unsafe in all pediatric age groups." Partial waivers could apply for specific age groups (FDA, "DRAFT Guidance for Industry: Recommendations for Complying With the Pediatric Rule (21 C.F.R. 314.55(a) and 601.27(a))," Center for Drug Evaluation and Research (CDER) and Center for Biologics Evaluation and Research (CBER), November 2000, http://www.fda.gov/downloads/Drugs/GuidanceCompliance RegulatoryInformation/Guidances/ucm072034.pdf).

[55] FDA, "Specific Requirements on Content and Format of Labeling for Human Prescription Drugs; Revision of "Pediatric Use" Subsection In the Labeling; Final rule," *Federal Register*, vol. 59, no. 238, December 13, 1994, pp. 64240-64250.

[56] Although market exclusivity is a characteristic of patent benefit, the FDA-granted exclusivity is not a patent extension; rather, it means that, during the six-month period, FDA would not grant marketing approval to another identical product (usually a generic). For more discussion of pharmaceutical patents and marketing exclusivity, see, for example, CRS Report RL33288, *Proprietary Rights in Pharmaceutical Innovation: Issues at the Intersection of Patents and Marketing Exclusivities*, by John R. Thomas.

[57] FDA, "Regulations Requiring Manufacturers to Assess the Safety and Effectiveness of New Drugs and Biological Products in Pediatric Patients; Final rule," *Federal Register*, vol. 63, no. 231, December 2, 1998, pp. 66632-66672.

[58] U.S. District Judge Henry H. Kennedy Jr. quoted in Marc Kaufman, "Judge Rejects Drug Testing on Children; Ruling Finds FDA Overstepped Authority in Forcing Pediatric Studies," *Washington Post*, October 19, 2002, p. A9.

In: Pediatric Drug Research and the FDA   ISBN 978-1-62257-729-3
Editors: K. Washington and J. Bennett   © 2013 Nova Science Publishers, Inc.

Chapter 2

PEDIATRIC RESEARCH: PRODUCTS STUDIED UNDER TWO RELATED LAWS, BUT IMPROVED TRACKING NEEDED BY FDA*

United States Government Accountability Office

WHY GAO DID THIS STUDY

In 2007, Congress reauthorized two laws, the Pediatric Research Equity Act (PREA) and the Best Pharmaceuticals for Children Act (BPCA). PREA requires that sponsors conduct pediatric studies for certain products unless the Department of Health and Human Services' (HHS) Food and Drug Administration (FDA) grants a waiver or deferral. Sponsors submit studies to FDA in applications for review. BPCA is voluntary for sponsors. The FDA Amendments Act of 2007 required that GAO describe the effect of these laws since the 2007 reauthorization. GAO (1) examined how many and what types of products have been studied; (2) described the number and type of labeling changes and FDA's review periods; and (3) described challenges identified by stakeholders to conducting studies. GAO examined data on the studies from the 2007 reauthorization through June 2010, reviewed statutory requirements, and interviewed stakeholders and agency officials.

---

* This is an edited, reformatted and augmented version of the Highlights of GAO-11-457, a report to congressional committees, dated May 2011.

WHAT GAO RECOMMENDS

GAO recommends that the Commissioner of FDA track applications during its review process and maintain aggregate data on applications subject to PREA. HHS agreed that better tracking of information is needed but disagreed with GAO's finding that it does not track applications. While FDA is able to identify the status of individual applications during its review, it has not maintained data that would allow it to better manage its review process.

WHAT GAO FOUND

At least 130 products—80 products under PREA and 50 under BPCA—have been studied for use in children since the 2007 reauthorization. However, FDA cannot be certain how many additional products may have been studied because FDA does not track and aggregate data about applications submitted under PREA that would allow it to manage the review process. FDA was unable to provide information about some applications that had been submitted to the agency that were subject to PREA. Recent improvements to FDA's data system might assist the agency in tracking future applications. Under PREA, FDA has granted most of the study waivers and deferrals requested by sponsors since the 2007 reauthorization. Under BPCA, FDA granted pediatric exclusivity—an additional 6 months of market exclusivity, which generally delays marketing of generic forms of the product—to the sponsors of 44 of the 50 drugs in exchange for conducting pediatric studies. Because BPCA is voluntary, sponsors may decline FDA's request for pediatric studies. Although BPCA includes provisions to encourage the study of drugs when sponsors have declined FDA's request, few drugs have been studied under these provisions.

Since the 2007 reauthorization, all of the 130 products with pediatric studies completed and applications reviewed under PREA and BPCA had labeling changes that included important pediatric information. The most commonly implemented labeling change expanded the pediatric age groups for which a product was indicated. The next most common type of labeling change indicated that safety and effectiveness had not been established in pediatric populations and provided a description of the study conducted. Additional labeling changes were recommended for products as a result of FDA's monitoring of adverse events associated with products after they had been approved for marketing. FDA officials said they need to complete their review of the application, including all studies, before they can reach agreement with the sponsor on labeling changes.

Stakeholders, including sponsors, pediatricians, and health advocacy organizations, described challenges faced by sponsors that could limit the success of PREA and BPCA. Those challenges included confusion about how to comply with PREA and BPCA due to a lack of guidance from FDA for changes to the laws from the 2007 reauthorization of PREA or BPCA. FDA officials explained that they mitigate this lack of guidance by discussing questions or concerns that sponsors have regarding their pediatric studies with sponsors throughout the process. An additional challenge sponsors described was a lack of economic incentives to study products with no remaining market exclusivity.

ABBREVIATIONS

BPCA	Best Pharmaceuticals for Children Act
DARRTS	Document Archiving, Reporting and Regulatory Tracking System
EU	European Union
FDA	Food and Drug Administration
FDAAA	Food and Drug Administration Amendments Act of 2007
FDAMA	Food and Drug Administration Modernization Act of 1997
FNIH	Foundation for the National Institutes of Health
HHS	Department of Health and Human Services
HIV	human immunodeficiency virus
NIH	National Institutes of Health
PAC	Pediatric Advisory Committee
PeRC	Pediatric Review Committee
PIP	paediatric investigation plan
PREA	Pediatric Research Equity Act
PPSR	Proposed Pediatric Study Request

May 31, 2011

The Honorable Tom Harkin
Chairman

The Honorable Michael B. Enzi
Ranking Member
Committee on Health, Education, Labor, and Pensions
United States Senate

The Honorable Fred Upton
Chairman
The Honorable Henry A. Waxman
Ranking Member
Committee on Energy and Commerce
House of Representatives

Congress and the Department of Health and Human Services' (HHS) Food and Drug Administration (FDA) have worked to increase the number of drug and biological products studied for use in children.[1] According to an article by FDA officials, researchers reported in 1999 that 81 percent of products used by children lacked sufficient information or labeling regarding pediatric use.[2,3] Products not labeled for pediatric use place children at risk of being exposed to ineffective or harmful treatment or receiving incorrect dosing. Since the late 1990s, Congress has passed laws to encourage or require product sponsors, typically the product's manufacturer, to conduct pediatric studies,[4] including the Pediatric Research Equity Act (PREA)[5] and the Best Pharmaceuticals for Children Act (BPCA).[6] As a result of these efforts, prior to the most recent reauthorizations of PREA and BPCA, pediatric studies resulted in approximately 250 labeling changes that added or clarified information on pediatric use of the product.

In 2007, as a part of the FDA Amendments Act of 2007 (FDAAA),[7] Congress reauthorized PREA and BPCA in order to increase the number of products studied for use in children. PREA requires that sponsors conduct pediatric studies for certain drug and biological products before they are marketed unless FDA grants a waiver or deferral for some or all pediatric studies. A waiver removes the requirement that some or all studies be completed, and a deferral allows the sponsor to conduct a study by a specified date after the product has been approved for marketing. BPCA, however, is voluntary for the sponsor; it authorizes FDA to provide an incentive of an additional 6 months of market exclusivity to product sponsors that conduct pediatric studies requested by FDA. This market exclusivity generally delays marketing of generic forms of the product and is known as pediatric exclusivity. Pediatric exclusivity can only be granted to those products that are "on-patent"—that is, those that have patent protection or market exclusivity.[8] BPCA also includes provisions (1) to allow for the funding of pediatric studies of on-patent drugs that the sponsor declined to study by the Foundation for the National Institutes of Health (FNIH)[9] and (2) to allow for the conduct of studies of "off-patent" products, which no longer have market exclusivity, through the National Institutes of Health (NIH).[10]

The results of pediatric studies conducted under PREA and BPCA are submitted to FDA in an application. The application includes pediatric study results and suggested labeling changes, among other things.[11] FDA reviews the application and works to come to agreement with the sponsor on labeling changes, which FDA then approves as part of its approval of the application.[12] PREA and BPCA require that one year after a product's labeling change is implemented, any adverse events reported for that product be reviewed. FDA may require additional labeling changes based on the adverse events.[13]

FDAAA required that we describe the effect PREA and BPCA have had on the study and labeling of drug and biological products for pediatric use.[14] To respond to the requirement in FDAAA that we report our findings to you no later than January 1, 2011, we briefed you on our findings on December 15, 2010. This report contains information we provided during that briefing as well as additional information in which you expressed interest. As discussed with the committees of jurisdiction, we (1) examine how many and what types of drug and biological products have been studied under PREA and BPCA since their 2007 reauthorization; (2) describe the number and type of labeling changes and FDA's review periods for reaching agreement on these changes for the drug and biological products for which studies have been completed since the 2007 reauthorization; and (3) describe challenges identified by stakeholders, including sponsors and other interested parties, to conducting pediatric studies. FDAAA also required that we describe efforts by FDA and NIH to encourage studies in neonates, which are children under the age of one month. We discuss these efforts in appendix I.

To examine how many and what type of drug and biological products have been studied under PREA and BPCA since their 2007 reauthorization, we reviewed FDA and NIH data on products studied in pediatric populations from the date of the 2007 reauthorization of PREA and BPCA through June 30, 2010, the most recent date for which data were available at the time of our analysis.[15] Specifically, we examined data on the number of products for which studies have been completed since the 2007 reauthorization. These studies were generally initiated prior to the reauthorization. We also examined data on the number of products for which studies were initiated since the 2007 reauthorization.[16] These studies are generally still ongoing. We compared FDA's procedures for tracking applications submitted under PREA to the standards described in the *Standards for Internal Control in the Federal Government*.[17] In examining FDA's procedures for tracking data, we examined the agency's ability to locate individual applications and its ability to track aggregate data about applications that would allow FDA to manage the review process, including the total number of applications subject to PREA, whether those applications were complete, and whether PREA applications included pediatric studies or requests for waivers or deferrals at the time of submission. We reviewed FDA data in order to determine the extent to which FDA waived or deferred the requirement for sponsors to submit studies under PREA. We also reviewed FDA data on the therapeutic areas, or conditions treated, for the products studied under PREA and BPCA. In addition, we interviewed officials from FDA, NIH, and FNIH.

To describe the number and type of labeling changes and FDA's review periods for reaching agreement on these changes for drug and biological products for which studies have been completed since the 2007 reauthorization, we analyzed FDA data on all pediatric labeling changes from the date of the 2007 reauthorization of PREA and BPCA through June 30, 2010, the most recent date for which the data were available at the time of our analysis.[18] Specifically, we determined the number and types of labeling changes that have been approved both as a result of pediatric studies and reported adverse events. In addition, we reviewed requirements in PREA and BPCA for reaching agreement on labeling changes and FDA documents on performance goals. We also interviewed FDA officials.

To describe challenges identified by stakeholders to conducting pediatric studies, we interviewed various stakeholders and reviewed articles written by some of these stakeholders. These stakeholders included representatives from five drug and biological product sponsors; three trade groups: the Pharmaceutical Research and Manufacturers of America, the Biotechnology Industry Organization,[19] and the Generic Pharmaceutical Association; and several health advocacy organizations, including the American Academy of Pediatrics, the National Organization for Rare Disorders, the Elizabeth Glaser Pediatric AIDS Foundation, the Tufts Center for the Study of Drug Development, the Institute for Pediatric Innovation, and the Pediatric Pharmacy Advocacy Group. In addition, we interviewed officials from FDA, NIH, and FNIH.

To assess the reliability of data that FDA and NIH provided, we interviewed agency officials. FDA and NIH officials described how they maintained data on pediatric studies conducted under PREA and BPCA, the resulting labeling changes, and pediatric adverse events. FDA generally maintained the information in separate files rather than centralized databases. To the extent possible, we looked for other sources of information to corroborate or provide perspective on the data FDA supplied. For example, we looked to data that is posted on FDA's Web site and compared it, when possible, to data provided directly by FDA. Although we found that FDA does not maintain certain data on the programs, we generally found the data that FDA maintains to be reliable for our purposes.

We conducted this performance audit from December 2009 through May 2011 in accordance with generally accepted government auditing standards. Those standards require that we plan and perform the audit to obtain sufficient, appropriate evidence to provide a reasonable basis for our findings and conclusions based on our audit objectives. We believe that the evidence obtained provides a reasonable basis for our findings and conclusions based on our audit objectives.

BACKGROUND

The FDA Modernization Act of 1997 (FDAMA) established pediatric exclusivity for sponsors that conducted pediatric studies for drugs.[20] In 1999, FDA implemented the Pediatric Rule, which required that sponsors include the results of pediatric studies when submitting certain new drug or biological product applications.[21] However, in 2002, the Pediatric Rule was declared invalid by a federal court.[22] In 2002, Congress reauthorized FDAMA's pediatric exclusivity provisions in BPCA, and in 2003, Congress codified much of the Pediatric Rule in PREA, requiring that pediatric studies be conducted and that the results of those studies be included in certain new drug or biological product applications. In September 2007, Congress reauthorized both PREA and BPCA as a part of FDAAA, and in March 2010, Congress extended pediatric exclusivity and applicable BPCA provisions to biological products as a part of the Patient Protection and Affordable Care Act.[23] PREA and BPCA are both set to expire on October 1, 2012.[24]

PREA

PREA requires that sponsors submit the results of pediatric studies in certain drug and biological product applications to FDA. Specifically, PREA applies to drug and biological product applications for any of the following: a new active ingredient, a new indication, a new dosage form, a new dosing regimen, or a new route of administration. In addition, PREA requires that pediatric studies be conducted for the indications described in the application—that is, the indications for which the sponsor plans to market the product—but not for any additional indications.

The 2007 reauthorization of PREA established the Pediatric Review Committee (PeRC), an internal FDA committee responsible for providing assistance in the review of pediatric study results and increasing the consistency and quality of such reviews across the agency.[25] The PeRC consists of approximately 40 FDA employees with a range of expertise, including pediatrics, biopharmacology, statistics, chemistry, legal issues, pediatric ethics, and others as pertinent to the pediatric product under review. FDA officials explained that the PeRC is divided into separate subcommittees for PREA and BPCA.

When a sponsor completes all of the required studies for a drug or biological product, it submits an application to FDA.[26] The application includes these study results and suggested labeling changes based on the pediatric studies' findings, among other things. If the pediatric studies have not been completed, the application must include a request for a waiver or deferral of the pediatric studies. PREA established certain criteria under which, at the sponsors' request, some or all of the required pediatric studies may either be deferred until a specified date after approval of the product's application or waived altogether by FDA.[27] FDA may also grant a deferral or waiver on its own initiative, under specified circumstances. For example, a study required under PREA may be deferred when additional data on the safety and effectiveness of the product in adults is needed before the product can be studied for use in children. If the sponsor requests a deferral, the product's application must include, among other things, a description of the planned pediatric studies and a time frame for completion. The study may be waived when it is determined to be impossible or highly impracticable, such as when the number of pediatric patients with a disease that may be treated with that product is too small to study. Sponsors may conduct multiple studies per product, such as separate studies for subsets of pediatric populations like infants, children, and adolescents. FDA may grant waivers or deferrals for only one type of study, such as in one pediatric age group, or FDA may grant waivers or deferrals for all pediatric studies of the product.

FDA's review of an application under PREA is part of the agency's broader review of the entire application. Once the sponsor submits its application, FDA directs the application to the agency's appropriate division to review the entire application, including all adult study results, the pediatric study results, and requests for a waiver or deferral. FDA may determine that the application is incomplete and more information is necessary from the sponsor. Generally, when this happens, FDA notifies the sponsor and waits to finish reviewing the application until the information is received. According to FDA officials, toward the end of FDA's review, the division provides requests for a waiver or a deferral and a summary of the relevant pediatric data to the PeRC for review. The PeRC provides recommendations on whether or not the pediatric portion of the application satisfies PREA requirements and whether to grant or deny a waiver or deferral. FDA then determines whether or not to approve the application. As a part of the review process, FDA is required by PREA to negotiate and reach an agreement with the sponsor on labeling changes based on pediatric studies within 180 days of the application's submission.[28] If FDA and the sponsor are unable to reach an agreement on labeling changes within 180 days, they are required by PREA to proceed to a formal dispute resolution process. The 2007 reauthorization of PREA provided FDA with authority to make labeling changes on its own initiative when a product has been studied for use in children, including when a study does not determine that the product is safe or effective in pediatric populations. Therefore, FDA can impose a labeling change unilaterally to describe FDA's determination about the study results in the event that the agency cannot reach agreement with the sponsor.

A sponsor can request that a drug or biological product that is required to be studied under PREA be studied under BPCA as well, to allow the sponsor of the product to be eligible to receive pediatric exclusivity.[29] According to FDA officials, the sponsor can make this request through a proposed pediatric study request (PPSR). If FDA agrees, it issues a formal written request to the sponsor that outlines, among other things, the nature of the pediatric studies that the sponsor must conduct in order to qualify for pediatric exclusivity. (See figure 1.) According to FDA officials, the pediatric studies requested under BPCA would generally also fulfill the PREA requirement; however, even if the sponsor does not complete the studies outlined in the BPCA written request, it is still required to complete any studies required under PREA. FDA officials said that pediatric studies conducted under BPCA are generally more extensive than those required under PREA. For example, the written request could include studies for indications in addition to those described by the sponsor in its application, such as those that are relevant to children.[30]

BPCA

Under BPCA, sponsors receive pediatric exclusivity as an incentive to conduct studies of drug and biological products for use in children.[31] The BPCA process formally begins when FDA determines that information related to the use of the product in a pediatric population may produce health benefits and issues a written request for pediatric studies to the sponsor of a product. Written requests may be issued for new, not previously marketed, drug or biological products or to products that are already on the market but still on-patent. FDA may issue a written request on its own initiative or after it has received and agreed to a PPSR from a sponsor to conduct a study under BPCA. The PeRC reviews all written requests and provides recommendations prior to their issuance to sponsors. According to FDA officials, in the written request, FDA may ask for more than one study of a single drug or biological product, such as studies for multiple indications or separate studies for different age groups, such as infants, children, and adolescents. BPCA requires that FDA take into account adequate representation of children of ethnic and racial minorities when developing written requests.[32] (See app. II for information on FDA's efforts to ensure the inclusion of racial and ethnic minorities in pediatric studies.) The sponsor must respond to FDA within 180 days of receiving the written request indicating whether the sponsor agrees to the request and, if so, when the pediatric study will be initiated. If the sponsor does not agree to the request, the sponsor must state the reasons for declining the request.

When the pediatric studies are complete, the sponsor submits the results to FDA in an application, which must include any suggested labeling changes resulting from the studies' findings. FDA recommends that the application be submitted 15 months prior to the end of the sponsor's market exclusivity for the product in order to be considered for pediatric exclusivity.[33] Once the sponsor submits its application, FDA is to review the sponsor's application in order to (1) determine whether or not to approve the application, (2) negotiate and reach an agreement with the sponsor on pediatric labeling changes, and (3) grant or deny pediatric exclusivity. FDA is to grant pediatric exclusivity if the study meets the conditions outlined in the written request, regardless of the study's findings. Specifically, in determining whether to grant or deny pediatric exclusivity, BPCA requires that FDA assess whether the studies fairly responded to the written request, were conducted in accordance with commonly accepted scientific principles and protocols, and were properly submitted.[34]

During FDA's review of the application, the PeRC may review a summary of relevant pediatric data from the application and provide recommendations to FDA on whether or not to grant pediatric exclusivity. FDA then determines whether or not to approve the application. In addition, if FDA and the sponsor are unable to reach an agreement on the labeling changes within 180 days, they are required by BPCA to proceed to the same formal dispute resolution process that exists for PREA.[35] The 2007 reauthorization of BPCA provided FDA with authority to make labeling changes on its own initiative when a product has been studied for use in children, including when a study does not determine that the product is safe or effective in pediatric populations. Therefore, FDA can impose a labeling change unilaterally to describe FDA's determination about the study results in the event that the agency cannot reach agreement with the sponsor.

BPCA includes provisions for the conduct of pediatric studies even if the sponsor declines the written request. If a sponsor declines a written request by FDA to study an on-patent drug or if a sponsor does not complete studies outlined in an accepted written request, FDA may refer the written request to FNIH if it determines that there is a continuing need for information relating to the use of the drug in the pediatric population. (See figure 2.) If FNIH is not able to fund all studies, BPCA requires that FDA consider whether to require the studies described in the written request under PREA.[36]

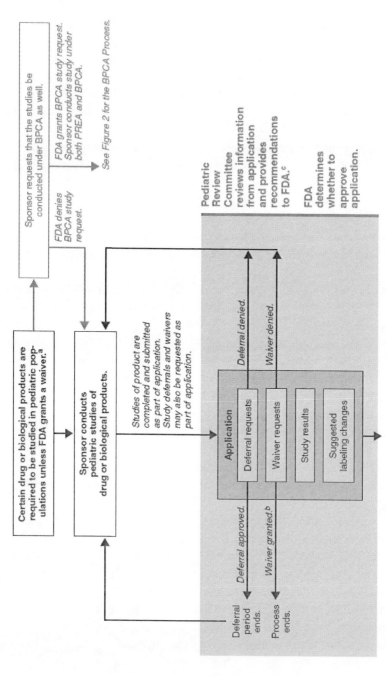

Source: GAO analysis of PREA requirements.

[a] PREA applies to drug and biological product applications for any of the following: a new active ingredient, a new indication, a new dosage form, a new dosing regimen, or a new route of administration.

[b] If a waiver is granted because the product would be ineffective and/or unsafe in children, such information must be included in the product's labeling.

[c] FDA provides requests for a waiver or a deferral and a summary of the relevant pediatric data to the Pediatric Review Committee for review.

[d] PREA requires that FDA and the sponsor enter dispute resolution if the labeling change is not agreed upon within 180 days of the application's submission.

Figure 1. PREA Process.

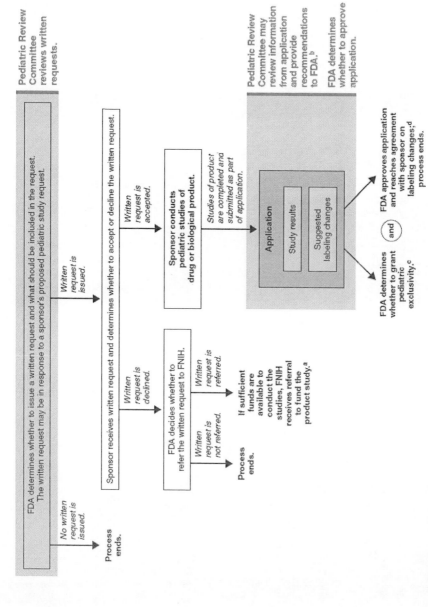

Source: GAO analysis of BPCA requirements.

Figure 2. BPCA Process for On-Patent Drug or Biological Products.

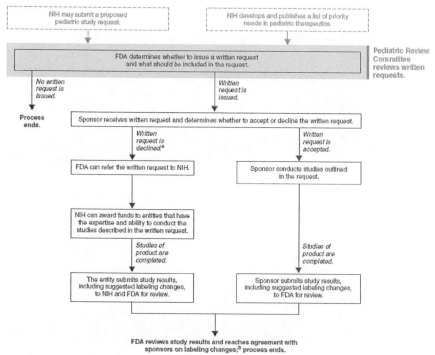

Source: GAO analysis of BPCA requirements.

[a] FDA also considers the written request to be declined if the sponsor does not respond to FDA within 30 days.

[b] BPCA requires that FDA and the sponsor enter dispute resolution if the labeling change is not agreed upon within 180 days of the submission of study results.

Figure 3. BPCA Process for Off-Patent Drug or Biological Products.

The process under BPCA for off-patent products differs from the process for on-patent products. To further the study of off-patent products, NIH— in consultation with FDA and experts in pediatric research—is required to develop and publish a list of priority needs in pediatric therapeutics, including products or indications that require study, every 3 years. NIH publishes this list on its Web site and in the *Federal Register*.[37] NIH may submit a PPSR to FDA for the study under BPCA of an indication of an off-patent product that is used for one of the pediatric therapeutic areas described on the NIH list of priority needs. FDA is then to determine whether to issue a written request in response to NIH's PPSR to all sponsors of the drug or biological product, including the product's original sponsor as well as any manufacturers of the generic product.[38] The PeRC reviews all written requests and provides recommendations prior to their issuance to sponsors. If a sponsor were to accept the written request, it would conduct the studies outlined in the request and then submit the study results and any suggested labeling changes to FDA for review. However, according to FDA officials, a sponsor has not accepted a written request to study an off-patent product since the 2007 reauthorization. Off-patent products do not qualify for pediatric exclusivity, so there are few financial incentives to conduct the studies.

Under the 2007 reauthorization of BPCA, if the sponsors were to decline or fail to respond to the written request for an off-patent product within 30 days, FDA can refer the written request to NIH to publish a request for proposals to conduct the studies. The sponsors of off-patent products are not required to respond to a written request. If within 30 days of FDA's issuance of the written request the sponsors do not accept or decline the request, FDA considers the request declined. NIH can then award funds— for example, through grants or contracts—to entities that have the expertise and ability to conduct the studies described in the written request. When these studies are complete, the entity that completed the studies is to submit the study results to NIH and FDA for review. For off-patent studies conducted by a sponsor or funded by NIH, FDA is to negotiate and reach an agreement with the product's sponsors on appropriate labeling changes resulting from the study findings within 180 days. (See figure 3.) As is the case with on-patent products studied under PREA and BPCA, if FDA is unable to reach an agreement on the labeling changes for an off-patent product within that time, FDA is required by BPCA to proceed to the formal dispute resolution process.

The Pediatric Advisory Committee

The Pediatric Advisory Committee (PAC) is an FDA advisory committee consisting of 14 voting members, who are appointed by the Commissioner of FDA and are knowledgeable in pediatric research, pediatric subspecialties, statistics, and/or biomedical ethics. The committee includes a representative from a pediatric health organization and a representative from a relevant patient advocacy organization. The PAC is responsible for reviewing reports of all adverse events reported for drug and biological products during a one-year period after a labeling change is made under PREA or BPCA and may review reports of pediatric adverse events in subsequent years. The committee makes recommendations to FDA on how to respond to the adverse events. PAC recommendations can include suggested labeling changes based on the adverse events, continued heightened monitoring of the product, the production or revision of a medication guide for consumers, or a return to routine monitoring of adverse events.

In addition, as required by PREA and BPCA, the PAC is to assist in FDA's dispute resolution if a proposed labeling change is not agreed upon by FDA and the sponsor within 180 days of submission of the application. If a labeling change enters dispute resolution, FDA is to first request that the sponsor make any labeling changes that FDA has determined to be appropriate. If the sponsor does not agree, FDA is to refer the matter to the PAC. The PAC is then to convene to review the results of the pediatric studies and provide recommendations to FDA on appropriate changes to the product's labeling, if any. FDA is then to consider the committee's recommendations and request that the sponsor make any labeling changes recommended by the PAC that FDA has determined to be appropriate. If the sponsor does not make the labeling change, FDA may deem the product misbranded.

Internal Control

The *Standards for Internal Control in the Federal Government* provides the overall framework for establishing guidelines for internal control that help government managers achieve desired objectives.[39] Internal control, which is synonymous with management control, comprises the plans, methods, and procedures used to meet missions, goals, and objectives. Internal control is not one event, but a series of actions and activities that occur throughout an entity's operations on an ongoing basis. The responsibility of good internal control rests with managers; they set the objectives, put the control mechanisms and activities in place, and monitor and evaluate these mechanisms and activities. Internal control includes a variety of activities such as ensuring effective information sharing throughout the organization and conducting ongoing monitoring of agency activities.

AT LEAST 130 PRODUCTS HAVE BEEN STUDIED IN NUMEROUS THERAPEUTIC AREAS UNDER PREA AND BPCA, BUT FDA DOES NOT KNOW IF ADDITIONAL PRODUCTS HAVE BEEN STUDIED

At least 130 products—80 products under PREA and 50 under BPCA—have been studied for use in children since the 2007 reauthorization. However, FDA does not know if additional products with pediatric studies are included in applications for which FDA reviews under PREA are incomplete. The products studied under PREA and BPCA represent a wide range of therapeutic areas. In addition, few drugs have been studied when sponsors have declined written requests.

FDA Cannot be Certain How Many Additional Products Have Been Studied under PREA; Most Requests for Waivers and Deferrals Have Been Granted

Since the 2007 reauthorization, at least 80 products have been studied under PREA, but FDA cannot be certain how many additional products may have been studied. FDA does not track and aggregate data about applications submitted under PREA until the PeRC has completed its review of information from the application. This generally occurs late in FDA's overall review of the application. Therefore, FDA was unable to provide information about some applications that had been submitted to the agency that were subject to PREA. For example, FDA officials could not provide aggregate data about the total number of applications, whether the applications were complete or incomplete, or whether the application included pediatric studies or requests for waivers or deferrals. Therefore, FDA could not be certain how many additional applications for which it has not yet completed its review under PREA include pediatric studies or requests for waivers or deferrals. This lack of data during the review process about applications subject to PREA, hampers FDA's ability to manage the review process, including whether FDA is meeting statutory requirements and whether the sponsor has complied with PREA's requirements for pediatric studies.

FDA officials said that approximately 830 applications submitted to FDA from September 27, 2007, through June 30, 2010, were subject to PREA, but could not provide a precise number. The PeRC has completed its review of information from 449 of these applications, 80 of which contained the results of pediatric studies. Fifty-nine were drugs and 21 were biological products. FDA could not provide information about the remaining 381 of the approximately 830 applications. Standards for internal control in the federal government provide that managers need certain data to determine whether they are meeting their agencies' missions, goals, and objectives.[40] This could include whether FDA is meeting PREA requirements and whether the sponsor has complied with PREA's requirements for pediatric studies. FDA officials explained that these 381 applications were submitted to FDA, and were under consideration in the relevant FDA division, but had not yet been reviewed by the PeRC, which advises FDA in its review of pediatric studies or requests for waivers or deferrals. FDA officials said that they could not provide any details about these applications without locating each application individually within the agency and reviewing it to determine whether it included pediatric studies or requests for waivers or deferrals, but stated that it is likely that most of the approximately 381 applications are for products that sponsors plan to market in adult indications and, therefore, would include a request for a deferral of the pediatric studies rather than completed pediatric studies. Although FDA officials could not say how many, they said that some of the approximately 381 applications may be incomplete and awaiting further review upon the sponsor's submission of additional materials, and that some of the applications may have been withdrawn by the sponsor. However, some of the applications could include the results of completed pediatric studies. Therefore, the total number of products with studies completed under PREA may be greater than 80.

HHS officials stated in its comments on a draft of this report that an update to the Document Archiving Reporting and Regulatory Tracking System (DARRTS), completed in May 2011, will provide them with the capability to include a code to indicate whether an application is subject to PREA.[41] However, the HHS comments do not state that this data system update would provide the internal controls necessary to track and aggregate data about applications that are currently under review, which would allow FDA to readily retrieve information to manage this program. In addition, HHS states that FDA does not currently plan to code applications retrospectively until they have ensured that there are available resources for such a project. Therefore, unless they do these things, FDA still will not know the status of the 381 applications, including whether the applications were complete or incomplete, or whether the applications included pediatric studies or requests for waivers or deferrals, until the review of those applications is compete.

FDA has granted a full or partial waiver or deferral to more than half of the applications that it has reviewed under PREA. According to FDA officials, of the 449 applications for which FDA has completed its review, FDA granted sponsors 237 waivers and 131 deferrals. FDA officials noted that, generally, most sponsors request deferrals of pediatric studies in the product's application rather than conduct the pediatric studies prior to submitting the product's application. FDA sometimes granted a full or partial waiver and a deferral to a single application, therefore a single application could be included in both totals. FDA officials could not provide additional information about the remaining 381 applications submitted to FDA during this period but not reviewed by the PeRC.

Waivers and deferrals were granted for multiple reasons. The reason most frequently cited for granting a waiver was that the drug or biological product studies were found to be impossible or highly impracticable. Waivers may be granted for this reason because, for example, the number of patients in that age group is too small. Most deferrals were granted because the product was ready to be approved for use in adults before pediatric studies had been completed. (See figure 4).

FDA officials also could not say how many studies are ongoing under PREA because the agency does not maintain a count of those studies. According to FDA, sponsors inform FDA of their plans for studies currently being conducted under PREA, but FDA does not aggregate data for these products until the sponsor completes the studies and the results are submitted to FDA for review.

50 Products Have Been Studied under BPCA since Its 2007 Reauthorization

Fifty products have been studied under BPCA from the 2007 reauthorization through June 30, 2010; FDA has reviewed applications for 50 of these products, none of which were biological products.[42] As noted earlier, sponsors submit studies to FDA as part of an application. According to FDA officials, FDA granted pediatric exclusivity to the sponsors of 44 of the 50 drugs.[43] Sponsors of five of the six drugs that did not receive exclusivity submitted only partial responses to the written request. FDA officials explained that FDA reviews study results as they are submitted, but does not make a pediatric exclusivity determination until it receives a full response to the written request. Therefore, although FDA completed its review of the applications, the pediatric exclusivity determination is pending the completion of the remainder of the studies FDA requested. FDA officials stated that FDA denied pediatric exclusivity for one of the products prior to the 2007 reauthorization because the studies completed by the sponsor did not meet the conditions of the written request.[44] Additionally, FDA officials told us that two additional drugs were studied between September 27, 2007, and June 30, 2010, but those studies were still undergoing FDA review.

Since the 2007 reauthorization, according to FDA officials, FDA has issued 37 written requests for on-patent drug and biological products to sponsors under BPCA, 25 of which originated from a PPSR submitted to FDA by the sponsor since the 2007 reauthorization of BPCA.[45] Sponsors agreed to 35 of the written requests. (See figure 5.) FDA officials stated that the sponsors completed studies for two of the written requests; studies for the remaining 33 written requests are ongoing.[46] The two other written requests were declined because the sponsors stated they would be unable to finish the studies by the completion date outlined in the written request.[47] FDA officials stated that FDA is in the process of determining whether there is a continuing need for the studies described in the two declined written requests. If so, FDA will refer these studies to FNIH pending the availability of sufficient funding at FNIH. We previously reported that about 19 percent of on-patent written requests were declined from 2002 though 2005.[48] Since the 2007 reauthorization, about 5 percent of written requests have been declined.

Drug and Biological Products Were Studied in a Wide Range of Therapeutic Areas

Drug and biological products were studied under PREA and BPCA for their use in the treatment of a wide range of diseases in children, including those that are common or life threatening. FDA categorized the products studied under PREA and BPCA into 16 broad categories of disease, which include endocrinology, infectious diseases, and oncology; at our request, FDA also categorized the products studied under PREA.[49] Some of the products studied were for the treatment of diseases that are common, including those for the treatment of asthma and allergies, while other products studied treat more life threatening diseases such as cancer or human immunodeficiency virus (HIV) infection. Additionally, some products studied were preventive vaccines. The largest numbers of products were studied for the treatment of neurological diseases and viral infectious diseases, with 23 products studied in each therapeutic area since the 2007 reauthorization. (See table 1.) This number includes both ongoing and completed studies that have been reviewed by FDA.

Few Drugs Have Been Studied When Sponsors Have Declined Written Requests

Since the 2007 reauthorization, none of the on-patent products for which written requests were declined or not completed by sponsors have been funded for study by FNIH. A provision under BPCA allows FDA to refer declined written requests for on-patent products to FNIH pending the availability of sufficient funding. However, according to FNIH representatives, FNIH does not have sufficient funding because it is no longer raising funds for the study of on-patent drugs under BPCA. Since the 2007 reauthorization, FNIH has partially funded the study of two on-patent drugs for which written requests were declined by sponsors or not completed, but NIH initiated and also partially funded those studies prior to the 2007 reauthorization. FDA has not referred any on-patent drugs to FNIH since the 2007 reauthorization of BPCA.

Since the 2007 reauthorization of BPCA, FDA has referred written requests for the study of two off-patent drugs that have been declined or not responded to by sponsors to NIH for funding. As of June 30, 2010, NIH initiated funding for the study of one of these two products, but NIH has not submitted any study results for this product to FDA. NIH has also funded 12 studies that are not product specific since the 2007 reauthorization of BPCA.

Prior to the reauthorization of BPCA, FDA referred 15 written requests for the study of off-patent drugs that were declined, or not responded to, by sponsors to NIH for funding. Of these 15 drugs, NIH funded the study of 10 of these drugs. As of June 30, 2010, NIH has submitted study results for two of these off-patent drugs to FDA; however, NIH has not yet completely satisfied the requirements of any written request for the study of an off-patent drug under BPCA.

Reasons studies were granted a waiver

Reasons studies were granted a deferral

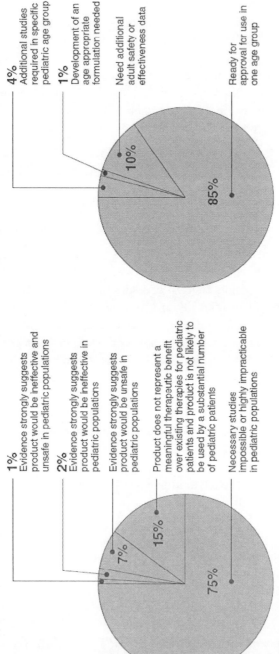

1%
Evidence strongly suggests product would be ineffective and unsafe in pediatric populations

2%
Evidence strongly suggests product would be ineffective in pediatric populations

Evidence strongly suggests product would be unsafe in pediatric populations

Product does not represent a meaningful therapeutic benefit over existing therapies for pediatric patients and product is not likely to be used by a substantial number of pediatric patients

Necessary studies impossible or highly impracticable in pediatric populations

4%
Additional studies required in specific pediatric age group

1%
Development of an age appropriate formulation needed

Need additional adult safety or effectiveness data

Ready for approval for use in one age group

Source: GAO analysis of FDA data.

Note: PREA contains categories of reasons for FDA to use when granting waivers and deferrals and the figure above reflects all of these reasons. However, FDA has never granted a waiver for the reason, "applicant can demonstrate that reasonable attempts to produce a pediatric formulation necessary for that age group have failed."

Figure 4. Reasons Applications Were Granted a Waiver or Deferral, September 27, 2007, through June 30, 2010.

Table 1. Products with Completed or Ongoing Pediatric Studies, Categorized by Therapeutic Area

Therapeutic areas	Examples of diseases associated with each therapeutic area	Number of products with completed or ongoing studies since the 2007 Reauthorizations of PREA and BPCA – September 27, 2007, through June 30, 2010		
		Ongoing (BPCA only)	Completed	
			PREA	BPCA
Addiction	Smoking cessation, maintenance of abstinence from alcohol in patients with alcohol dependency.	0	0	0
Analgesia/anesthesiology/ anti-inflammatory	Anesthesia; pain	4	3	1
Cardiovascular disease	Congestive heart failure; hypertension	2	1	4
Dermatology	Dermatitis; skin and skin structure infections	0	6	1
Endocrinology/metabolism	Diabetes Mellitus; obesity	1	5	8
Gastroenterology	Crohn's Disease; ulcers	1	2	6
Hematology/coagulation	Deep vein thrombosis (thromboembolism)	1	4	1
Infectious disease (viral)	Hepatitis B virus, human immunodeficiency virus (HIV) infection and/or prophylaxis of HIV infection in exposed neonates	5	7	11
Infectious disease (non viral)	Malaria; pneumonia (bacteremic)	2	4	1
Medical Imaging	Myocardial perfusion imaging; Cardiac imaging	1	1	1

Table 1. (Continued)

Therapeutic areas	Examples of diseases associated with each therapeutic area	Number of products with completed or ongoing studies since the 2007 Reauthorizations of PREA and BPCA – September 27, 2007, through June 30, 2010		
		Ongoing (BPCA only)	Completed	
			PREA	BPCA
Neurology	Adolescent schizophrenia; depression/major depressive disorder	5	7	11
Oncology	Brain tumors and other solid tumors; hematologic tumors	8	1	1
Ophthalmology	Conjunctivitis; intraocular pressure	1	10	0
Other therapeutic areas	Symptoms associated with common cold and influenza;	0	5	1
Pulmonary	Allergic Rhinitis; asthma	2	12	3
Preventive vaccine[a]	Vaccines	0	12	0

Source: FDA.

Note: A product may be used to treat more than one therapeutic area. For the purposes of this table, a product is counted once for each therapeutic area it is used to treat. Therefore, the number of products with completed or ongoing studies by therapeutic area is greater than the total number of products with completed or ongoing studies.

[a] Preventive vaccines are not considered by FDA to be therapeutic products but rather, are considered to be vaccines to prevent disease caused by specific bacteria or viruses. We included them for the purpose of providing a full outline of the types of products studied under PREA.

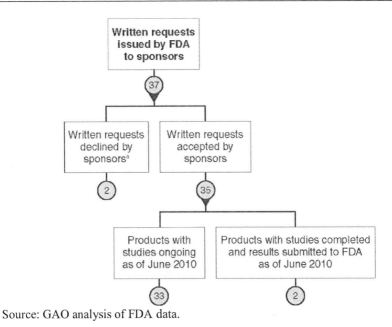

Source: GAO analysis of FDA data.

Figure 5. Written Requests Issued for On-Patent Drug and Biological Products, September 27, 2007, through June 30, 2010.

NIH does not receive appropriations specifically to fund studies for products under BPCA. NIH officials said that NIH institutes and centers spend a total of $25 million annually on BPCA activities, which are coordinated by the Eunice Kennedy Shriver National Institute of Child Health and Human Development. NIH officials have said that when FDA refers a written request for the study of a product under BPCA to NIH, NIH must determine if it is feasible to initiate funding for the product's studies. This determination depends on the availability of funding and the feasibility of conducting the necessary pediatric studies.[50] NIH officials stated that funding a clinical trial with approximately 200 patients costs an average of almost $10 million over 5 years. In addition, NIH annually spends $4.5 million of this $25 million it spends on BPCA activities on the contract for NIH's BPCA data coordinating center.

ALL PRODUCTS WITH COMPLETED PEDIATRIC STUDIES HAD LABELING CHANGES, AND FDA'S GOALS OFTEN DIFFER FROM THE PREA REQUIREMENT FOR REACHING AGREEMENT ON LABELING CHANGES

All of the drug and biological products with pediatric studies completed and applications reviewed since the 2007 reauthorization had labeling changes that included important pediatric information. FDA's goals for the time it takes to review applications often differ from the requirement in PREA for reaching agreement on labeling changes with the sponsor.

All Products with Completed Pediatric Studies since the 2007 Reauthorization Had Labeling Changes That Included Important Pediatric Information

All of the 130 drug and biological products with studies completed and applications reviewed by FDA since the 2007 reauthorization had labeling changes.[51] As a point of comparison, in the 9 years prior to the 2007 reauthorization, 256 products had pediatric study-related labeling changes agreed upon by FDA and the product's sponsor. (See table 2.) In addition, we previously reported that not all products studied under BPCA had labeling changes.[52] According to FDA officials, instances in which there were no labeling changes for products studied prior to the 2007 reauthorization were generally due to study results that did not establish that the products were safe and/or effective in children. The 2007 reauthorizations of PREA and BPCA provided FDA with authority to make labeling changes on its own initiative when a product has been studied in children, including when a study does not determine that the product is safe or effective in pediatric populations.

The labeling changes for drug and biological products studied under PREA and BPCA reflected important pediatric information. FDA categorizes labeling changes into one or more of nine categories, and each drug or biological product can have more than one category of labeling change. These categories illustrate the important pediatric information provided in labeling changes, ranging from providing new or enhanced safety information to inserting a boxed warning for pediatric populations. Since the 2007 reauthorization, the most commonly implemented labeling change expanded the pediatric age groups for which a product was indicated. There were 99 instances of this type of labeling change. (See table 3.) For example, a labeling change for a drug treating gastroesophageal reflux disease extended the approved indication from adults only to pediatric patients 5 years of age and older. In addition, 28 labeling changes indicated that, though a study was conducted, safety and effectiveness had not been established in pediatric populations. For example, pediatric studies on a drug meant to treat osteogenesis imperfecta, a genetic disorder commonly known as brittle bone disease, did not show a reduction in the risk of bone fracture in children. Therefore, the drug's labeling was changed to describe the study conducted and indicate that safety and effectiveness were not established in pediatric populations.

Since the 2007 reauthorization, the PAC reviewed the adverse events reported for 74 drug and biological products and recommended additional labeling changes for 17 of those 74 products.[53] (See figure 6.) As of June, 30, 2010, FDA reported that it had approved 7 of the 17 PAC-recommended labeling changes. Of the remaining 10 PAC-recommended labeling changes, FDA was still considering whether to approve 5 labeling changes and had decided not to approve 5 labeling changes. According to FDA, these five PAC-recommended labeling changes were not approved because, after further review of the adverse events, FDA determined that labeling changes were not necessary. Reasons underlying these determinations include an insufficient link between the reported adverse events and the product and the presence of confounding factors, such as other preexisting conditions that may have contributed to the adverse event.

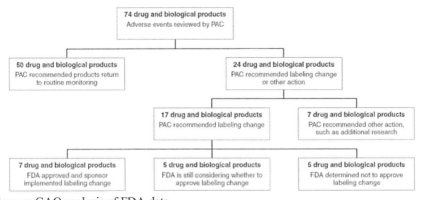

Source: GAO analysis of FDA data.

Figure 6. Pediatric Advisory Committee (PAC) Recommendations for Drug and Biological Product Adverse Events, September 27, 2007, through June 30, 2010.

Table 2. Number of Drug and Biological Products That Had Pediatric Labeling Changes as a Result of Studies Conducted under PREA or BPCA

	PREA abeling changes		BPCA labeling changes		Pediatric Rule labeling changes[a]		
	Drugs	Biological products	Drugs	Biological products[b]	Drugs	Biological products	Total
Pre 2007 Reauthorization (Oct. 1998 – Sept. 26, 2007)	72	0	136	0	48	0	**256**
Post 2007 Reauthorization (Sept. 27, 2007 – June 30, 2010)	59	21	50	0	0	0	**130**
Total							**386**

Source: GAO analysis of FDA data.

[a] The Pediatric Rule went into effect in 1999, but a federal court declared the Pediatric Rule invalid in October 2002. In 2003 Congress codified much of the Pediatric Rule in PREA.

[b] BPCA did not apply to biological products until the Patient Protection and Affordable Care Act extended pediatric exclusivity to biological products.

FDA's Goals Often Differ from the PREA Requirement for Reaching Agreement on Labeling Changes

FDA's performance goal for the time it takes for FDA to review most PREA applications often differs from PREA's requirement for the time FDA is to take to reach agreement with the sponsor on labeling changes.[54] According to FDA officials, the agency cannot adequately consider and agree upon a labeling change until it completes its review of an application. FDA is required by both PREA and BPCA to negotiate and reach agreement with the sponsor on labeling changes based on pediatric study results within 180 days of submission of the application. If FDA is unable to reach agreement with the sponsor, it is required to enter the labeling change dispute resolution process. FDA's review of suggested labeling changes is part of a broader review— FDA's review to determine whether or not to approve the application—for which it has specific performance goals that include time periods within which it seeks to review applications.[55] Under these performance goals, applications are classified as either priority or standard, depending on the characteristics of the application, and FDA has committed to completing its review of 90 percent of priority applications within 180 days of submission and 90 percent of standard applications within 300 days of submission. BPCA requires that applications submitted under BPCA that propose a labeling change, which are all BPCA applications, receive priority status. Therefore, all BPCA applications have been subject to 180-day review. However, according to FDA officials, only a subset of applications subject to PREA requirements—those that provide major advances in therapy or new therapies—receive priority status. All other applications submitted under PREA are to be reviewed within the standard 300 days of submission.

Table 3. Number of Labeling Changes for Drug or Biological Products by Category of Change, September 27, 2007, through June 30, 2010

Categories of labeling changes for drug or biological products[a]	PREA		BPCA		Total
	Drugs	Biological products	Drugs	Biological products[b]	
Expanded pediatric age groups approved in the label, including the addition of new pediatric indications	50	19	30	0	99
Provided new or enhanced pediatric safety information	10	4	8	0	22
Determined that safety and effectiveness was not established in pediatric populations and added a description of the study conducted	3	2	23	0	28
Provided information on a specific change or adjustment to the pediatric dosing	3	0	2	0	5
Provided label for a new pediatric formulation of an existing drug or biological product	2	0	6	0	8
Provided original labeling, including pediatric information, for a new active ingredient that was never before marketed in the United States	3	0	0	0	3
Inserted a boxed warning for pediatric populations	0	0	1	0	1
Provided pharmacists with detailed step-by-step instructions on how to prepare formulations for pediatric populations	0	0	4	0	4
Provided details on dosing differences between pediatric and adult populations due to pharmacokinetic differences	0	0	1	0	1

Source: GAO analysis of FDA data.

[a] Each labeling change can be categorized as more than one category of change.

[b] BPCA did not apply to biological products until the Patient Protection and Affordable Care Act extended pediatric exclusivity to biological products.

For priority applications, FDA's goal to complete its review of the application within 180 days is consistent with the labeling change requirements of PREA and BPCA since the two review periods—the application review goal and the labeling change review period—are both 180 days. However, for PREA applications subject to standard review, which includes most PREA applications, the goal and required review period are different. FDA's goal to complete its review of the application within 300 days differs from PREA's requirement to reach agreement on labeling changes within 180 days. FDA officials acknowledged that the agency has generally not agreed upon labeling changes within the required 180 days for PREA applications subject to standard review. However, as noted previously, FDA could not account for 381 applications submitted to the agency under PREA, making it difficult for FDA to determine whether it is meeting either the requirements of PREA or the agency's goals for these applications. FDA has never initiated the labeling change dispute resolution process. According to FDA officials, the agency has been able to reach agreement with sponsors on labeling changes without needing to initiate this process.

STAKEHOLDERS IDENTIFIED AGENCY GUIDANCE, UNCERTAINTY ASSOCIATED WITH REAUTHORIZATION, AND LACK OF ECONOMIC INCENTIVES AS POTENTIAL CHALLENGES TO CONDUCTING PEDIATRIC STUDIES

Stakeholders whom we interviewed described several challenges to conducting pediatric studies. One challenge stakeholders, including sponsors, identified was confusion about how to comply with PREA and BPCA due to a lack of current guidance from FDA. FDA officials acknowledged that the most recent PREA guidance is draft guidance from 2005 and that the most recent BPCA guidance was revised in 1999. FDA has not provided guidance for changes to the laws from the 2007 reauthorization for PREA or BPCA. FDA officials stated that they plan to publish updated guidance on PREA and BPCA. However, they have no timeline for when they plan to do so. FDA explained that officials can discuss study timelines and questions or concerns sponsors may have regarding their study submissions throughout the process.

Stakeholders said another challenge is that reauthorizations of PREA and BPCA have led to uncertainty given the time required to conduct studies. They said that since PREA and BPCA are subject to reauthorization every 5 years, some of the statutory requirements for studies could change while studies are under way or as they are being planned; therefore, there is uncertainty as to the requirements that will apply when they conduct studies.[56] Two sponsors stated this uncertainty makes it difficult to know what will be involved in developing products for use in children over the long term, which makes it difficult to plan studies. For the 50 drugs for which FDA has completed its review since the 2007 reauthorization of BPCA, the average amount of time from when FDA issued a written request through when it completed its review of a drug's study results was 6 years. Based on this experience, PREA and BPCA would be reauthorized during the course of a drug or biological product study, possibly changing the requirements with which the sponsors must comply. For example, the 2007 BPCA reauthorization added the requirement that sponsors submit applications at least 9 months before the end of the product's market exclusivity.[57]

Another challenge identified by stakeholders is complying simultaneously with the U.S. laws, PREA and BPCA, and the European Union's (EU) Paediatric Regulation.[58] (See app. III for a description of the Paediatric Regulation.) Stakeholders stated that it is common for a sponsor to seek approval of a drug or biological product in both the EU and the United States simultaneously, making it necessary for the study to comply with PREA or BPCA and the Paediatric Regulation if the sponsor wants to market the drug in the United States and in the EU. For example, in the EU, the sponsor submits a plan for the study of a product in pediatric populations that must be approved by the European Medicines Agency before studies are conducted. Stakeholders stated, in the United States, sponsors do not have formal contact with FDA regarding their pediatric study design for studies submitted under PREA until they submit completed study results to FDA. Therefore, sponsors cannot be certain that studies done to comply with the Paediatric Regulation will meet FDA requirements.

Finally, stakeholders told us that the lack of economic incentives presents a challenge to sponsors' willingness to conduct pediatric studies voluntarily, as under BPCA. Stakeholders, including industry representatives, told us that sponsors are reluctant to conduct studies for drug and biological products that are nearing the end of their market exclusivity or are off-patent because there is no economic benefit associated with conducting these studies. Once a drug or biological product is off-patent, the sponsor cannot receive pediatric exclusivity for conducting pediatric studies. Stakeholders told us that these drug and biological products are among the least likely to be studied in pediatric populations. Given the lack of economic incentive, a provision in

BPCA gives NIH the responsibility of awarding funds to entities that have the expertise and ability to conduct studies of off-patent drug and biological products. However, stakeholders reported that NIH's ability to conduct these studies is limited due to a lack of resources devoted to this type of research.

CONCLUSION

At least 130 drug and biological products have been studied in pediatric populations under PREA and BPCA in a variety of therapeutic areas since the laws' 2007 reauthorization, resulting in important labeling changes. While this illustrates the laws' success in facilitating pediatric studies, we found that FDA did not have procedures in place to track and aggregate data about applications subject to PREA until the PeRC completed its review of the pediatric information included in the applications. Even though an application subject to PREA cannot be considered complete unless it contains pediatric study results or a request for a waiver or deferral, FDA has not been tracking whether these are included until information from the application is reviewed by the PeRC. According to FDA officials, the PeRC generally reviews information about pediatric studies submitted as part of the application near the end of FDA's application review process. Because of the timing of this review, FDA staff managing the review process cannot be certain how many applications that have been submitted to the agency are subject to PREA, how many of those applications include pediatric studies, or how many applications include requests for waivers or deferrals, until FDA has almost completed its review of the entire application. FDA's review of applications can last 300 days or more in some cases, depending on the specific attributes of the application.

FDA lacks an important internal control that would allow it to manage its review process to ensure that the agency and sponsors are meeting the law's requirements and that FDA is meeting its own mission, goals, and objectives during the period of its review of the application. Because several of the requirements of PREA and internal FDA goals focus on the amount of time FDA takes to conduct a review or make a decision and because some products studied under PREA may already be on the market for adult use, it is imperative that FDA have this information available to it throughout the review process. FDA's inability to track how long it has had an application or whether or not an application includes pediatric study results until after the PeRC has completed its review could delay the dissemination of important pediatric study results.

RECOMMENDATION FOR EXECUTIVE ACTION

We recommend that the Commissioner of FDA move expeditiously to track applications upon their submission and throughout its review Executive Action process and maintain aggregate data, including the total number of applications that are subject to PREA and whether those applications include pediatric studies.

AGENCY COMMENTS AND OUR EVALUATION

We provided a draft of this report to the Secretary of HHS for comment. In its comments, HHS noted that PREA and BPCA have been very successful in generating important pediatric labeling of drugs and biological products. HHS also agreed that better tracking of pediatric labeling and other information is needed and expressed the hope that future improvements in its databases will allow the agency to easily identify all pediatric studies contained in all applications. HHS acknowledged that such improvements could permit health care providers, the public, and other stakeholders to conduct more interactive and thorough searches for pediatric studies, indications, and other information relevant to pediatric patients.

In its comments, HHS disagreed with our finding that FDA does not have a system to track data about applications under PREA. The comments note that the FDA Center for Biologics Evaluation and Research has a specific code in its Regulatory Management System for Biologics Licensing Application that allows it to track PREA-filed applications for biological products. HHS describes the FDA Center for Drug Evaluation and Research's process for tracking applications using DARRTS and suggests that DARRTS allows FDA to track the status of any application at any given time.

However, our recommendation is not based on FDA's ability to determine the status of individual applications, but rather its lack of aggregate data on applications that are subject to PREA during its review of the applications so as to be able to better manage its review process. We clarified our discussion of our findings in this area and the wording of our recommendation. As discussed in this report, FDA was unable to determine how many of the applications that had been filed with the agency since PREA's 2007 reauthorization were subject to PREA. We had initially requested this information in an effort to provide context to some of the other information that we reported about FDA's implementation of PREA. FDA was able to report that approximately 830 applications were subject to PREA, but was unable to provide a precise number. Since this was considerably more than the 449 applications that had been reviewed by the PeRC, we sought additional information about the status of these applications. In response to our request, FDA officials explained that the agency did not maintain this information and that determining the status of these applications would require that they engage in a labor intensive manual process that would require an extensive investment of FDA resources and would take months to complete. We believe that FDA's lack of aggregate data about an important program designed to enhance the safety of drug and biological products for use in children is inconsistent with sound internal controls because it does not provide FDA officials with the information they need to effectively manage the program to ensure that the review process is being implemented in accordance with statutory and other requirements until the process is almost complete.

In its comments, HHS states that in May 2011, FDA made an improvement to DARRTS that was not in place during the time of our review. HHS states that the improvement will allow FDA to better track future applications that are subject to PREA. However, the comments do not state whether the improvement will allow FDA to determine during its review process whether applications include studies or requests for waivers or deferrals. While it remains unclear what data will be readily available to FDA officials as they manage this program, FDA's efforts to improve its tracking of applications are consistent with the goal of our recommendation and should enable it to better track future applications. HHS's comments state that FDA hopes to include enhanced information about applications in DARRTS retrospectively, but notes that the agency will have to ensure that there are available resources for such a project. Therefore, DARRTS will not include this improved data for applications that are currently undergoing review.

HHS states that FDA maintains data about completed studies under PREA on its Web site. However, this data is compiled and placed on FDA's Web site after FDA's review of the applications is complete. Our finding and recommendation address the lack of data that FDA has available about PREA applications during the review process, which can last 300 days or more.

We incorporated changes to the report to address HHS's comments about FDA's ability to track applications and incorporated technical comments as appropriate.

Marcia Crosse

Director, Health Care

APPENDIX I. INCLUSION OF NEONATES IN DRUG AND BIOLOGICAL PRODUCT STUDIES

The Food and Drug Administration (FDA) Amendments Act of 2007 required that we describe the efforts made by FDA and the National Institutes of Health (NIH) to encourage that studies be conducted in children 4 weeks old or less, also known as neonates. This appendix describes the efforts of FDA and NIH to encourage studies in neonates and their efforts to ensure that those studies are safe. We also describe the number of products with completed and ongoing studies in neonates since the 2007 reauthorization of the Pediatric Research Equity Act (PREA) and the Best Pharmaceuticals for Children Act (BPCA).[59] In addition, we describe the challenges to increasing the inclusion of neonates in pediatric drug studies identified by physicians.

To describe the efforts of FDA and NIH to encourage studies in neonates, we interviewed FDA and NIH officials and examined FDA and NIH data to summarize the number of pediatric drug studies being conducted in neonates under PREA and BPCA. To assess the reliability of the data FDA and NIH provided, we interviewed agency officials. FDA and NIH officials described how they maintained data on pediatric studies, and the resulting labeling changes conducted under PREA and BPCA. We found the data reliable for our purposes. We also reviewed literature on studies conducted in neonates and barriers to these studies. We interviewed stakeholders including representatives from three trade groups, the Pharmaceutical Research and Manufacturers of America, the Biotechnology Industry Organization[60] and the Generic Pharmaceutical Association. We also interviewed health advocacy organizations, including the American Academy of Pediatrics, the National Organization for Rare Disorders, the Elizabeth Glaser Pediatric AIDS Foundation, the Tufts Center for the Study of Drug Development, the Institute for Pediatric Innovation, and the Pediatric Pharmacy Advocacy Group.

To describe the challenges to increasing the inclusion of neonates in pediatric drug studies identified by physicians, we convened two panel discussions; we were assisted in convening one of the panels by the American Association of Pediatrics and another by a director of neonatology at a large research hospital. The panelists in both instances were physicians who conducted pediatric drug studies in neonates. We also interviewed FDA and NIH officials.

FDA's efforts to encourage the inclusion of neonates in pediatric drug studies and its efforts to ensure that those studies are safe and effective have been focused on including neonates in its written requests. However, in some instances FDA has requested neonates' inclusion but not required it. Since the 2007 reauthorization of BPCA, FDA has issued four written requests to drug sponsors that have mentioned neonates specifically.[61] FDA required the inclusion of neonates in the written request for the study of one of the four drugs. FDA's written requests for three other drugs asked for the inclusion of neonates in the study; however, the sponsors of these products had the option of not including neonates in the studies. The sponsors will inform FDA as to whether they included neonates in the studies when they submit completed study results to FDA for review.

Sponsors have submitted completed studies to FDA that have included neonates for nine products—eight drugs and one biological product— since the 2007 reauthorization; FDA has reviewed all study results and labeling changes have been made reflecting neonate information for all of the products.[62] Seven of these studies were submitted under BPCA; two were submitted under PREA.

NIH has funded studies under BPCA for five drugs that have included neonates. These studies were initiated before the 2007 reauthorization, but are ongoing. Additionally, NIH has conducted several activities under BPCA to ensure the safety and effectiveness of drugs in neonates, including neonates that are premature. These activities include the 2009 co-funding of a large scale study of the diagnosis and treatment of hypotension in premature infants, funding of a study to determine outcome measures for chronic lung disease in premature infants, and the development of a small volume sampling technique for neonates with congenital heart disease.

FDA officials explained that a limited number of the studies conducted under PREA have included neonates because PREA only requires that pediatric studies be conducted for the indication described on the drug application, which is typically applicable to adults and older pediatric populations that would not apply to neonates.[63] Additionally, PREA provides sponsors with the option to request that required pediatric studies be waived by FDA when there is a valid reason. For some applications, FDA has agreed to waive studies after it has determined that including neonates in a drug study may be impossible or highly impracticable due to safety or ethical concerns.

FDA and NIH officials explained that they face challenges in increasing the inclusion of neonates in pediatric studies under BPCA. BPCA authorizes FDA to provide an incentive of an additional 6 months of market exclusivity, known as pediatric exclusivity, to product sponsors that conduct pediatric studies requested by FDA. FDA officials explained that they have been granting pediatric exclusivity for the study of products in children older than one month, so it is difficult to have manufacturers go back and do the study in neonates because it may be difficult for them to receive additional pediatric exclusivity.[64] FDA officials told us that the neonate population has diseases that are very different from other pediatric populations and that there are limited tools that can be used to study these diseases. FDA and NIH officials told us that there are also ethical issues that arise when working with this population that create a barrier. Based on our review of the literature, we found there is an ethical issue concerning whether neonates are a vulnerable population that should not be enrolled in trials where there may be increased risk to their health.

The physicians that we spoke with as a part of our two panels explained that they encounter numerous challenges to conducting studies in neonates. One challenge the panelists described is obtaining informed consent from the parents, which is required for the neonate to be enrolled in a study. For example, one panelist stated that because the mother may be medicated from her delivery it may be difficult to obtain consent from her. One panelist stated that he encounters families for which English is their second language and he may need them to review and understand a complex 10- to 12- page study outline that is written in English. The panelist explained that while his hospital provides doctors who speak another language and may communicate in that language for families for which English is a second language, they may encounter another challenge if the family is not able to read in their native language.

The panel explained that there are also scientific challenges to conducting studies in neonates. One scientific challenge is that the amount of blood in neonates is extremely limited. However, blood must be drawn to determine proper dosing of the products being tested, requiring doctors to do needle pricks to obtain blood from the neonate. These pricks are in addition to the pricks that must be done to monitor the health of the neonate and there may not be enough blood to test for both proper dosing and to monitor the neonate's health. The panel went on to explain that the outcomes of the study must be observed in the neonate between 3 to 5 years after the study. This level of monitoring is costly to the sponsor and can be an economic disincentive to conducting studies in neonates. The panel also explained that neonates are heterogeneous—there can be a significant difference in a neonate born at 23 weeks than a neonate that is 40 weeks—and any study designed to include them must account for this, making it difficult to generalize the study results.

Panelists said that another challenge to increasing the inclusion of neonates in studies involves FDA, stating that FDA sometimes seems to be creating barriers rather than working to include neonates in studies. For example, they said that FDA has required that a product be proven safe and effective for adults before it can be studied in neonates; however the panelists stated that because neonates often have illnesses that are specific to their age and condition, this requirement does not make sense. Furthermore, one panelist stated that she believed that FDA did not have enough neonatologists on staff to assist in preparing written requests. She also stated that it is important that study designs that include neonates be reviewed by neonatologists and not general pediatricians because neonatologists understand the issues that must be confronted in the neonatal intensive care unit. FDA's Pediatric Review Committee, which reviews written requests and determines whether waivers and deferrals should be granted, has about 40 members. However, FDA officials we interviewed said that there is only one neonatologist on the Committee.[65] Additionally, the FDA officials stated that there are three neonatologists in the two FDA divisions that review pediatric studies. FDA officials said that they do not have the resources to hire additional neonatologists.

APPENDIX II. INCLUSION OF ETHNIC AND RACIAL MINORITY PARTICIPANTS IN PEDIATRIC DRUG STUDIES

The Food and Drug Administration Amendments Act of 2007 (FDAAA) requires that FDA consider the adequate representation of children of ethnic and racial minorities when issuing written requests to sponsors to conduct pediatric studies for a product under the Best Pharmaceuticals for Children Act (BPCA).[66,67] It is important to include minorities in pediatric studies because proteins, metabolizing enzymes, and genetic traits can differ among races and ethnicities. We previously reported that these differences may result in a product having adverse or unexpected side effects for users depending on their race or ethnicity.[68] To examine how FDA considered the representation of ethnic and racial minority participants in product studies conducted under BPCA, we reviewed the 37 written requests that FDA issued to sponsors from the time of the 2007 reauthorization of BPCA on September 27, 2007 through June 30, 2010.

FDA issued guidance in 2005 on the collection of race and ethnicity data in clinical trials recommending that sponsors use a standardized approach developed by the Office of Management and Budget to report the race and ethnicity of study participants.[69] FDA's 2005 guidance recommends, rather than requires, that sponsors use the specified categories because participants' racial and ethnic data may not be able to be collected in some instances and because the specified categories may not be sufficient or appropriate for some studies. For example, when studies are conducted outside of the United States, the recommended categories may not adequately describe the racial and ethnic groups in foreign countries.

FDA has issued 37 written requests to sponsors for the study of on-patent products under BPCA, since the 2007 reauthorization. In these 37 written requests, FDA asked that sponsors include information on the representation of ethnic and racial minorities for all participants using the standardized categories specified in agency guidance when responding to written requests.[70] In all but two of the 37 written requests, FDA also requested that if the sponsor chose to use other categories, the sponsor obtain FDA's agreement on the use of alternate categories.

APPENDIX III. PEDIATRIC DRUG AND BIOLOGICAL PRODUCT STUDIES IN THE EUROPEAN UNION AND THE UNITED STATES

The European Union's Paediatric Regulation for the development of drug and biological products in pediatric populations was implemented in January of 2007 in order to facilitate the development of, and improve the availability of information on, products for use in children.[71] The European Union's Paediatric Regulation is similar to laws on pediatric studies in the United States, some form of which has been in existence since 1997.[72] To describe the European Union's Paediatric Regulation for drugs and biological products, we examined European Medicines Agency literature, the Paediatric Regulation, United States laws, and additional sources regarding United States and

European Union pediatric laws and regulations. We also interviewed FDA officials.

The European Union's Paediatric Regulation

The Paediatric Regulation requires sponsors to submit a plan for the study of a product in pediatric populations, known as a paediatric investigation plan (PIP), early in the development of a new product. PIPs are required to include the sponsor's proposed timing and methods for conducting pediatric studies in all age groups. Sponsors must submit PIPs to the Paediatric Committee, which was created by the Paediatric Regulation. Sponsors submit to the Paediatric Committee through the European Medicines Agency. The Paediatric Committee reviews the PIP and determines whether to agree or refuse the study plan. The PIP is a binding agreement between the sponsor and the European Medicines Agency, but can be modified as necessary. The Paediatric Regulation allows for the agency to either defer pediatric studies until the product has been studied in adults or waive the studies altogether in certain circumstances.[73] The Paediatric Committee is responsible for granting or denying deferrals and waivers. When studies are deferred, the sponsor must still submit a PIP that includes details on the pediatric studies that will be conducted and when those studies will begin, but when studies are waived, the requirement to submit a PIP is also waived.

Once a new product is ready to be marketed, the sponsor submits a marketing authorization application to the European Medicines Agency that must include, among other things, the results of pediatric studies conducted in accordance with the PIP or proof that a waiver or deferral of the pediatric studies was granted.[74] If the sponsor has conducted studies in compliance with the PIP, it is entitled to a six-month extension of the product's market exclusivity. Additional information on the Paediatric Regulation can be found on the European Medicines Agency website.[75]

European Union and United States Collaboration

The European Union and the United States collaborate by exchanging information in order to ensure that pediatric studies are conducted in a scientifically rigorous and ethical manner and that pediatric patients are not exposed to duplicative studies. Stakeholders stated that it is common for a sponsor to seek approval of a drug or biological product in both the EU and the United States, making it necessary for a sponsor to comply with both the EU and United States' pediatric study processes if it wants to market the drug in both locations. In addition, the European Medicines Agency and the FDA communicate and collaborate to share information such as the status of current studies, written requests, PIPs, waivers and deferrals, study results, safety concerns, and other topics. According to FDA's Web site, from August 2007 to March 2009, the European Medicines Agency and the FDA discussed 144 products.[76] This communication and information sharing between the European Medicines Agency and the FDA takes place through monthly teleconferences and by using a secure electronic system.

End Notes

[1] Biological products are derived from living sources (such as humans, animals, and microorganisms), unlike drugs, which are chemically synthesized. Biological products include blood, vaccines, allergenic products, certain tissues, and cellular and gene therapies. See 42 U.S.C. § 262(i).

[2] See D. K. Benjamin Jr., et al, "Safety and Transparency of Pediatric Drug Trials," *Archives of Pediatrics & Adolescent Medicine*, vol. 163, no. 12 (2009).

[3] Drug or biological product "labeling" includes all labels and other written, printed, or graphic materials on any container, wrapper, or materials accompanying the product. 21 U.S.C. § 321(k), (m).

[4] A drug or biological product sponsor is the person or entity who assumes responsibility for the marketing of a new product, including responsibility for complying with applicable laws and regulations.

[5] 21 U.S.C. §§ 355c, 355d.

[6] 21 U.S.C. § 355a; 42 U.S.C. § 284m.

[7] Pub. L. No. 110-85, §§ 401-404, 501-503, 121 Stat. 823, 866-90 (2007).

[8] See 21 U.S.C § 355a(n)(1)(B); 42 U.S.C. § 284m. For purposes of this report, we refer to drug and biological products that have patent protection or market exclusivity as "on-patent" and those whose patent protection or market exclusivity has ended as "off-patent". This is the same terminology typically used by government agencies to describe the exclusivity status of a product under BPCA.

[9] FNIH is an independent, nonprofit corporation. The majority of funds that FNIH receives are from the private sector. FNIH funds are used for a variety of purposes, including awards to researchers to conduct studies related to BPCA. See 42 U.S.C. § 290b.

[10] NIH is an agency within HHS and is comprised of 27 institutes and centers, each with a specific research agenda.

[11] For products studied under PREA or BPCA, sponsors generally submit new drug applications, supplemental new drug applications, biologics license applications, or supplemental biologics license applications to FDA. Before a drug or biological product can be marketed in the United States, the sponsor must submit a new drug application or a biologics license application to FDA containing data demonstrating the safety and efficacy of the product. After a product is marketed, sponsors submit supplemental new drug applications or supplemental biologics license applications to support proposed changes to a product's

labeling, a new dosage form or strength of the product, a new patient population or intended use, or changes to the way the product is manufactured. See 21 U.S.C. § 355 (drugs); 42 U.S.C. § 262 (biological products).

[12] Although the product studied might be new to the market and, therefore, its labeling would be new and not a change, FDA characterizes the agreement on labeling as a "labeling change" under PREA and BPCA.

[13] FDA uses the term "adverse event" to refer to any untoward medical event associated with the use of a drug or biological product in humans.

[14] Pub. L. No. 110-85, § 404, 121 Stat. 823, 875-76.

[15] The 2007 reauthorization of PREA and BPCA was enacted and went into effect on September 27, 2007.

[16] FDA generally reports data to the public on the number of studies conducted under PREA and BPCA, but for the purposes of this report we report on the number of products studied. Since sponsors can conduct multiple studies per product, the number of products studied will be less than the total number of studies conducted. We counted each application submitted by the sponsor to FDA as one product. We counted the following types of applications: new drug applications, supplemental new drug applications, biologics license applications, and supplemental biologics license applications. For studies conducted under BPCA, FDA reports studies by active moiety, or molecule responsible for the physiological or pharmacological action of the drug substance, rather than product. A single moiety could be active in multiple products, such as different strengths of the same dosage form, or a moiety could be present in different dosage forms such as a lotion form and a tablet form. Therefore, because we analyzed the number of products studied, not moieties studied, we may report a different number of products studied than the moieties reported by FDA. For the purposes of our report when we refer to products studied, we are referring to products whose studies have been completed and for whom FDA has completed the application review for the product. In addition, for the purposes of our analyses, we considered all products with biologics license applications as biological products.

[17] See GAO, *Standards for Internal Control in the Federal Government*, GAO/AIMD-00-21.3.1 (Washington, D.C.: November 1999). Internal control comprises the plans, methods, and procedures used to meet missions, goals, and objectives.

[18] We also reviewed data on labeling changes that occurred prior to the 2007 reauthorization in order to provide context to the total number of labeling changes that have occurred as a result of laws providing for pediatric studies, some form of which has been in existence since 1997.

[19] The Biotechnology Industry Organization assisted us in convening a panel discussion that included representatives from four drug and biological product sponsors.

[20] Pub. L. No. 105-115, § 111, 111 Stat. 2296, 2305-09.

[21] 63 Fed. Reg. 66,632-66,672 (Dec. 2, 1998).

[22] Implementation of the Pediatric Rule prompted a lawsuit against FDA by the Association of American Physicians and Surgeons, the Competitive Enterprise Institute, and Consumer Alert, which claimed that FDA acted outside of its authority in issuing the Pediatric Rule. In 2002, the court ruled that FDA exceeded its authority in issuing the rule and declared the rule invalid. Association of American Physicians & Surgeons v. FDA, 226 F. Supp.2d 204 (D.D.C. 2002).

[23] Pub. L. No. 111-148, § 7002(g)(1), 124 Stat. 119, 819-20 (to be codified at 42 U.S.C. § 262(m)).

[24] 21 U.S.C. §§ 355a(q), 355c(m).

[25] See 21 U.S.C. § 355d.

[26] Applications that are subject to PREA are submitted to FDA for approval and undergo a broad application review process that, in addition to reviewing pediatric studies, reviews the results of adult studies and determines whether the application demonstrates that the product is safe and effective for the indicated population.

[27] 21 U.S.C. § 355c(a)(3), (4). If a waiver is granted because the product would be ineffective and/or unsafe in children, such information must be included in the product's labeling.

[28] 21 U.S.C. § 355c(g)(1). FDA's review of proposed labeling changes is part of its review of the application. Application review is subject to its own specified time frames. Under the 2007 reauthorization of the prescription drug user fee program as a part of FDAAA, FDA committed to performance goals related to the review of drug applications and biologics license applications, including time frames within which it seeks to review applications. See Pub. L. No. 110-85, § 101(c), 121 Stat. 823, 825 (2007). The performance goals are identified in letters sent by the Secretary of Health and Human Services to the Chairman of the Senate Committee on Health, Education, Labor, and Pensions and the Chairman of the House Committee on Energy and Commerce and are published on FDA's Web site. Each fiscal year, FDA is required to submit a report on its progress in achieving those goals and future plans for meeting them. See 21 U.S.C. § 379h-2(a). Under these performance goals, drug and biological product applications are classified as either priority or standard, and FDA committed to completing its review of 90 percent of priority applications within 180 days of submission and 90 percent of standard applications within 300 days of submission. Applications submitted under PREA may be either priority or standard, depending on the characteristics of the applications.

[29] For the purposes of this report, we report data on products studied in this manner under BPCA. FDA reports data on these products in a separate category of products studied under both PREA and BPCA.

[30] These additional indications are often referred to as "off-label" indications.

[31] In March 2010, the Patient Protection and Affordable Care Act extended pediatric exclusivity and applicable BPCA provisions to biological products. See Pub. L. No. 111-148, § 7002(g)(1), 124 Stat. 119, 819-20 (codified at 42 U.S.C. § 262(m)).

[32] In a 2003 report, we recommended FDA specify in its written requests that sponsors use the standard racial and ethnic categories described in FDA's January 2003 draft guidance. See GAO, *Pediatric Drug Research: Food and Drug Administration Should More Efficiently Monitor Inclusion of Minority Children*, GAO-03-950 (Washington, D.C.: Sept. 26, 2003), p. 18.

[33] BPCA requires that FDA make the determination that the sponsor has met the study requirements outlined in the written request 9 months prior to the end of the drug or biological product's market exclusivity. 21 U.S.C. § 355a(b)(2), (c)(2). FDA officials explained that because BPCA provides the agency with 180 days to review the study results, FDA recommends that the sponsor submit its results 15 months prior to the end of its market exclusivity. See 21 U.S.C. § 355a(d)(3).

[34] 21 U.S.C. § 355a(d)(3). Pediatric exclusivity applies to all approved uses of the drug or biological product, not just those studied in children. Therefore, if the studies find that the product is not safe for use by children, the product will still receive pediatric exclusivity— that is, extended market exclusivity—for the adult uses of the product.

[35] 21 U.S.C. § 355a(i)(2). FDA's review of proposed labeling changes is part of its review of the application. BPCA requires that all applications submitted under BPCA that propose a labeling change receive priority status and be subject to FDA's performance goals for priority products, under which FDA seeks to complete its review of 90 percent of priority applications within 180 days of submission. See 21 U.S.C. § 355a(i)(1). PREA does not contain this requirement.

[36] Under a provision in BPCA added by the 2007 reauthorization, if FNIH does not have sufficient funds, FDA is required to consider whether to require a sponsor of an on-patent drug already on the market to conduct pediatric studies under PREA. FDA may require studies in this manner if FDA finds that the product is used for a substantial number of pediatric patients for the labeled indication and adequate pediatric labeling could confer a benefit on pediatric patients, the product would represent a meaningful therapeutic benefit over existing therapies for pediatric patients for a labeled indication, or the absence of

adequate pediatric labeling could pose a risk to pediatric patients. 21 U.S.C. § 355a(n), § 355c(b). FDA has never invoked this provision to require studies of on-patent products for which sponsors have declined written requests.

[37] Prior to the 2007 reauthorization, instead of a list of therapeutic areas, BPCA required NIH to develop an annual list of specific drugs that the agency determined were in need of study in children.

[38] See 42 U.S.C. § 284m(c).

[39] GAO

[40] GAO

[41] According to FDA, DARRTS is intended to be a flexible, integrated, fully electronic workflow tracking and information management system to receive, log, track, assign, process, and manage official submissions with internal and external stakeholders. FDA is releasing DARRTS in stages. The first version was released in January 2006. Updates to the system, which incorporate additional types of FDA data into DARRTS, have been periodically implemented.

[42] Studies for all but two of these products were initiated prior to the 2007 reauthorization.

[43] Thirty-one of the 50 drugs with completed and reviewed studies were required to be studied under PREA, but sponsors requested and received written requests for the products to be studied under BPCA, as well.

[44] FDA officials explained that one product was denied pediatric exclusivity prior to the 2007 reauthorization because the sponsor did not enroll the number of participants in the study that was required by the written request. We included this product in our group of products studied since the 2007 reauthorization because FDA conducted further analysis of the product using the submitted results to try to determine the safety and effectiveness of the product's use in children. This additional information was used for a labeling change after the 2007 reauthorization.

[45] According to FDA officials, sponsors have submitted 64 PPSRs to FDA since the 2007 reauthorization. Twenty-five of these PPSRs resulted in a written request. FDA officials said that some of the written requests issued after the 2007 reauthorization were issued in response to PPSRs submitted to FDA before the 2007 reauthorization. However, FDA officials noted that there was a flaw in the system that tracks PPSRs and, therefore, they could not state with certainty the exact number of PPSRs that the agency had received.

[46] The two completed studies are also counted as two of the 50 products with completed and reviewed studies under BPCA. The written requests that prompted the studies were issued and the studies have been completed since the 2007 reauthorization.

[47] According to FDA officials, the timelines outlined in the written request are based on the statutory requirements outlined in BPCA.

[48] See GAO, *Pediatric Drug Research: Studies Conducted under Best Pharmaceuticals for Children Act*, GAO-07-557 (Washington, D.C.: March 22, 2007), p.12.

[49] FDA does not generally categorize the drug and biological products studied under PREA. FDA provided the therapeutic areas for products with completed studies under PREA in response to our request.

[50] When determining the feasibility of conducting the necessary pediatric studies, NIH considers the frequency and severity of the condition, the availability of a patient population, and the capability of researchers to conduct the studies.

[51] PREA requires that if a product is granted a waiver due to strong evidence that the product would be ineffective and/or unsafe in children, such information must be included in the labeling. 21 U.S.C. § 355c(a)(4)(D). Since the 2007 reauthorization, an additional 17 products received waivers that resulted in a labeling change on this basis.

[52] See GAO

[53] PREA and BPCA require that one year after a product's labeling change is implemented, the PAC review any adverse events reported for that product. In subsequent years, FDA will

determine whether to refer any additional pediatric adverse events reported for that product to the PAC for review.

[54] An application includes, among other things, suggested labeling changes based on study findings.

[55] Under the 2007 reauthorization of the prescription drug user fee program as part of FDAAA, FDA committed to performance goals related to the review of drug applications and biologics license applications, including time frames within which it seeks to review applications. See Pub. L. No. 110-85, § 101(c), 121 Stat. 823, 825 (2007). The performance goals are identified in letters sent by the Secretary of Health and Human Services to the Chairman of the Senate Committee on Health, Education, Labor, and Pensions and the Chairman of the House Committee on Energy and Commerce and are published on FDA's website. Each fiscal year FDA is required to submit a report on its progress in achieving those goals and future plans for meeting them. See 21 U.S.C. § 379h-2(a).

[56] However, the 2007 reauthorization of PREA and BPCA provides that certain studies pending before the date of the 2007 reauthorization are subject to prior versions of PREA and BPCA. See Pub. L. No. 110-85, §§ 402(b), 502(a)(2), 121 Stat. 823, 875, 885 (2007).

[57] BPCA requires that FDA make the determination that the sponsor has met the study requirements outlined in the written request 9 months prior to the end of the drug or biological product's market exclusivity. 21 U.S.C. § 355a(b)(2), (c)(2). FDA officials explained that because BPCA provides the agency with 180 days to review the study results, FDA recommends that the sponsor submit its results a minimum of 15 months prior to the end of its market exclusivity. See 21 U.S.C. § 355a(d)(3).

[58] The Paediatric Regulation is a single law that both requires sponsors to conduct studies as well as provides a 6-month exclusivity extension.

[59] See 21 U.S.C. §§ 355a (BPCA), 355c (PREA), 355d (PREA); 42 U.S.C. § 284m (BPCA).

[60] The Biotechnology Industry Organization assisted us in convening a discussion that included representatives from four of the drug sponsors.

[61] Since the 2007 reauthorization, FDA has issued 37 written requests for on-patent drug and biological products to sponsors under BPCA.

[62] Sponsors submitted incomplete study results to FDA for studies that included neonates for two other products. FDA has informed each sponsor that it will discontinue its review until the sponsor has completed the studies and resubmitted them.

[63] From September 27, 2007, through June 30, 2010, sponsors have submitted completed studies to FDA that have included neonates for two products under PREA.

[64] Under very narrow circumstances specified in BPCA, a drug may be eligible for additional pediatric exclusivity for a supplemental application. See 21 U.S.C. § 355a(g)(1).

[65] Our review of the Pediatric Review Committee roster found that there are two neonatologists on the committee as of April 15, 2010.

[66] See Pub. L. No. 110-85, § 502(d)(1)(A), 121 Stat. 823, 879 (2007) (codified at 21 U.S.C. § 355a(d)(1)(A)).

[67] BPCA encourages sponsors to conduct pediatric studies requested by the Food and Drug Administration in drug and biological products that are new or already on the market but still under patent protection by offering the sponsors 6 months of additional market exclusivity, known as pediatric exclusivity. See 21 U.S.C. § 355a; 42 U.S.C. § 284m. In March 2010, Congress extended pediatric exclusivity and applicable BPCA provisions to biological products as part of the Patient Protection and Affordable Care Act. Pub. L. No. 111-148, § 7002(g)(1), 124 Stat. 119, 819-20 (to be codified at 42 U.S.C. § 262(m)).

[68] See GAO, *Pediatric Drug Research: Food and Drug Administration Should More Efficiently Monitor Inclusion of Minority Children*, GAO-03-950 (Washington, D.C.: Sept. 26, 2003.

[69] See FDA, *Guidance for Industry: Collection of Race and Ethnicity Data in Clinical Trials* (Rockville, MD: Sept. 2005).

[70] FDA's 2005 guidance recommends that sponsors use the United States Office of Management and Budget's categories for data on race which are: American Indian or Alaska Native,

Asian, Black or African American, Native Hawaiian or other Pacific Islander, and White. Office of Management and Budget's categories for data on ethnicity are: Hispanic or Latino, and Not Hispanic or Latino.

[71] Regulation (EC) 1901/2006 of 12 December 2006 on Medicinal Products for Paediatric Use, 2006 O.J. (L 378) 1; Regulation (EC) 1902/2006 of 20 December 2006 amending Regulation 1901/2006 on Medicinal Products for Paediatric Use, 2006 O.J. (L 378) 20.

[72] See 21 U.S.C. §§ 355a (Best Pharmaceuticals for Children Act), 355c (Pediatric Research Equity Act), 355d (Pediatric Research Equity Act); 42 U.S.C. § 284m (Best Pharmaceuticals for Children Act).

[73] Waivers of pediatric studies may be granted to sponsors when products: (1) are likely to be ineffective or unsafe in part or all of the pediatric population; (2) are intended for conditions that occur only in adult populations; or (3) do not represent a significant therapeutic benefit over existing treatments for pediatric patients.

[74] The requirement also applies to applications for a new indication, new pharmaceutical form, or new route of administration.

[75] www.ema.europa.eu/

[76] This is the most recent data available from FDA's Web site. See www.fda.gov/Science Research/SpecialTopics/PediatricTherapeuticsResearch/ucm106621.h tm

INDEX